D0403839

Praise for *Finding Your Way to Change*

"This brilliant book guides you through a journey of discovery in that most intimate and difficult relationship—the one with yourself. Stories of others who have made the trek illustrate the challenges of being stuck in a problem that seems intractable, the way through the mire, and the joy of emerging on the other side. The book offers not only the promise of change, but also the ability to sustain it."
—David B. Rosengren, PhD, Prevention Research Institute

"The method in this book can fuel the fire of change and help you move from despair to positive action. The exercises are wonderful. The book helped me think differently about a dilemma in my own life, and I found myself reading parts of it to a friend who came to me for advice."
—Theresa B. Moyers, PhD, Department of Psychology and Center on Alcoholism, Substance Abuse, and Addictions, University of New Mexico

"A friend suggested that I read this book when she learned I was considering a career change. It provided me with a useful toolkit for considering what I want to do next, based on my own deep-seated interests and visions of my professional life. The concepts and techniques are easy to grasp. Previously, I tried to make difficult decisions by listing the pros and cons—this book offers a more sophisticated and thoughtful approach."   —John F.

"If you've ever said to yourself, 'I really want to change, but I just can't seem to do it,' you need to read this excellent book. Dr. Zuckoff knows that there are powerful forces within us that can sabotage our good intentions and best-laid plans. He gives you practical, scientifically grounded tools to help you understand why you're spinning your wheels and how to productively work through it."
—Henny Westra, PhD, CPsych, Department of Psychology, York University, Canada

WITHDRAWN

FINDING YOUR WAY TO CHANGE

FINDING
Your Way to
CHANGE

How the Power of
MOTIVATIONAL INTERVIEWING
Can Reveal What *You* Want
and Help You Get There

Allan Zuckoff, PhD
with Bonnie Gorscak, PhD

Foreword by William R. Miller and Stephen Rollnick

THE GUILFORD PRESS
New York   London

© 2015 The Guilford Press
A Division of Guilford Publications, Inc.
370 Seventh Avenue, Suite 1200, New York, NY 10001
www.guilford.com

The information in this volume is not intended as a substitute for consultation
with healthcare professionals. Each individual's health concerns should be
evaluated by a qualified professional.

Printed in the United States of America

This book is printed on acid-free paper.

Last digit is print number: 9   8   7   6   5   4   3   2   1

Library of Congress Cataloging-in-Publication Data

Zuckoff, Allan, 1960–
    Finding your way to change : how the power of motivational interviewing can
reveal what you want and help you get there / Allan Zuckoff, with Bonnie Gorscak.
        pages cm
    Includes index.
    ISBN 978-1-4625-2040-4 (paperback)—ISBN 978-1-60918-064-5 (cloth)
    1. Change (Psychology)   2. Motivation (Psychology)   3. Interviewing—
Psychological aspects.   I. Gorscak, Bonnie.   II. Title.
    BF637.C4Z83 2015
    158.1—dc23

                                                                    2014050371

To Gerry Zuckoff (1931–2014),
mother and mother-in-law,
loved and missed by us both

Contents

Foreword   ix

Acknowledgments   xi

A Note on Authorship   xiii

PRELUDE: *Considering Change*   I

I. You Don't Have to Change

1. *Being Ambivalent*   I3

2. *The Pressure Paradox*   35

3. *The Other Side of the Pressure Paradox*   59

II. Do You Want to Change? Can You Change?

FIRST INTERLUDE: *The Language of Change*   85

4. *Exploring the Importance of Change to You* 93

5. *Exploring Your Confidence for Change*   118

6. *Exploring Your Personal Values*   139

SECOND INTERLUDE: *Ready or Not?*   162

III. **Finding YOUR Way to Change**

THIRD INTERLUDE: *Planning for Change*   175

7. *Developing Your Plan*   181

8. *Revisiting, Revising, and Regrouping*   213

9. *The Far Side of Change*   231

APPENDIX. *The History and Science*   249
                     of Motivational Interviewing

Resources   257

Index   259

About the Authors   264

Purchasers of this book can download
and print forms from the online supplement
at *www.guilford.com/zuckoff-forms*.

Foreword

We introduced motivational interviewing (MI) over 30 years ago as an approach to be used in conversations between clients and their counselors. Many studies since then have found it to be an effective way of helping people change. Our original efforts with this counseling style were directed at people facing difficult life challenges like changing their health habits or getting free from an addiction. We found that deep listening helped people as they faced why and how they might change.

Now here is a book, *Finding Your Way to Change*, that addresses a new question: Can you use some of the same insights and practical ideas on your own to support important changes? There are solid links between the worlds of counseling and self-help that this book highlights. One example is the idea of ambivalence, or uncertainty about whether or not to change. It's something that we emphasize in counseling, and an understanding of this internal conflict is the focus of the first chapter. Another link is that being gentle and accepting of yourself can serve as a foundation for change. When you feel unacceptable, it's very hard to change; but when you take the pressure off and accept your situation, it becomes possible.

Based on the principles and practices of MI, this book is designed to help you get unstuck from ambivalence and move ahead with positive changes you might choose to make in your life. It gathers up-to-date knowledge and insights from MI into the world of self-help, offering useful ideas without falling prey to the hyperbole that is so common in self-help books. The authors do not dispense quick tricks or promise to give you something that you lack. Rather, they help you find that which you already have within you and draw out your own motivations for and wisdom about change.

Change in the face of ambivalence is a very common human predicament. We applaud the authors for translating the science and practice of MI into a useful skills-based book for anyone who wants to find his or her way to change.

WILLIAM R. MILLER, PhD
Emeritus Distinguished Professor
    of Psychology and Psychiatry
University of New Mexico

STEPHEN ROLLNICK, PhD
Honorary Distinguished Professor
Cochrane Institute of Primary Care
    and Public Health
School of Medicine, Cardiff University
Cardiff, Wales

· · · · · · · · · · ·

Acknowledgments

From the time I was introduced to motivational interviewing (MI) as a therapist seeing people with addiction and mental health problems in a public outpatient clinic, I have been fascinated by its deceptive simplicity and often profound impact. The opportunity to share what I have learned beyond the confines of the therapy office or training room feels like both a gift and a culmination.

I am most deeply grateful to William R. Miller and Stephen Rollnick, not only for MI and their unceasing efforts to improve it, but for exemplifying the values of affirming presence, generosity, gentleness in the face of conflict, and humility that animate their creation.

The members of the Motivational Interviewing Network of Trainers (MINT) share a dedication to a humane way of being and a spirit of international pluralism that reflect and amplify the virtues of MI's founders. Through annual forums and year-round electronic communications they have challenged and furthered my thinking about MI and given me a sense of community unlike any I have known. In particular, as the writing of this book unfolded, Sandy Downey offered feedback and support that made a difference. And I must thank my fellow members of the MINT Board of Directors, who taught me just how much can be accomplished through egoless teamwork.

Research on new counseling approaches not only puts innovations to the test; it immerses clinician-researchers in the approach they are testing, resulting in a deeper understanding of its workings and a greater ability to convey that understanding to others. I have been fortunate to collaborate in MI-related studies with a stellar collection of researchers, including

Holly Swartz, Nancy Grote, Blair Simpson, Mary Amanda Dew, Melanie Gold, Katherine Shear, Ellen Frank, and Dennis Daley.

I was given the chance to write this book because David Rosengren, the author of *Building Motivational Interviewing Skills*, thought I was the right person for the job and told his editor at The Guilford Press so. I had a number of reasons to be grateful to David before that, but this one topped them all.

David's editor, Kitty Moore, and developmental editor, Chris Benton, provided editorial guidance combining sharp insight, practical wisdom, encouragement, and much-needed patience. They made this book possible, and they made it better. So did Theresa Moyers, whose review of the manuscript, in true MI form, affirmed its strengths and highlighted places where there was room for growth.

My brother, Mitchell Zuckoff, is a professor of journalism, an award-winning reporter, and a best-selling author. Yet, for me, these accomplishments pale in comparison with what he has achieved as a father, husband, and man of integrity. He has written that no matter how old we get, he will always be trying to impress his older brother. I hope he knows that I look up to him as much as he has ever looked up to me.

It is no accident that my brother and I both became teachers. Sid Zuckoff, our father and model, showed us how important it is to take ideas seriously and to help others learn. He also taught us, through his actions, to give selflessly and unstintingly to the people we love. His careful proofreading of the manuscript was just the smallest illustration of this principle.

Alex Zukoff, my son, has grown from a sweet and startlingly psychologically minded child into a young man of passion, intelligence, creativity, and kindness. He is the embodiment of the observation that we learn as much from our children as they learn from us. He gave my life new meaning when he entered this world, and he continues to make the whole thing worthwhile.

Two women bookend my life. My mother, Gerry Zuckoff, was unswervingly dedicated to the happiness and well-being of her children, her husband, and just about every other person she ever came into contact with. She was an extraordinary woman and the reason I had both the ability and the desire to become a psychotherapist. My collaborator in work and life, Bonnie Gorscak, moves through the world seeing things in people that others don't. Her empathic and accepting way of being with people is coupled with a relentless drive to solve the mysteries of their motivations and behavior. When I met her I knew I had met my match, and then some. Marrying her was the best decision I ever made.

ALLAN ZUCKOFF

A Note on Authorship

It is traditional for authors to say in their acknowledgments that they could not have completed their work without the support of their spouse. Well, in this instance, that is no mere platitude.

The voice that speaks to you in this book expresses the understanding of motivational interviewing I have developed through almost 20 years of practice, teaching, and research. All of the writing in that authorial voice was done by me.

But it is one thing to describe the nature of ambivalence about change, what keeps people stuck, and how people can change if they choose to, and to develop MI-based activities to help readers explore and resolve their ambivalence; it is another to create a group of ambivalent people and imagine how they would respond to those activities. The latter is the special gift of my coauthor, Bonnie Gorscak. We thought about who the five people accompanying the reader should be, and together we developed their histories and the dilemmas they were facing. (All five companions are composites of clients we have worked with. All the other people who appear in this book—with the exception of the story of Bonnie and Kylie on pages 139–140 and my own story on page 231, which are described as they happened—are based on real people with whom I have worked, but any identifying elements of their stories and characteristics have been changed to protect their privacy.) Bonnie also drafted the companions' responses to most of the book's activities for my revision. As a result, it is literally true that I could not have completed this book without her.

• • • • • • • • • • •

Prelude

Considering Change

Something in your life has become an issue for you.

- It might be a habit—one you want to eliminate or one you want to cultivate.
- It could be a situation—one you're thinking about getting out of or one you're wondering about getting into.
- It might be a pattern—how you relate to others or try to get what you want out of life.

Whatever the issue is, it's not going away (although you might be wishing it would!). Maybe that's because someone else wants you to change, although you're not sure you need to. Maybe *you* believe something has to be done but can't decide what. Perhaps you know what you should do, but making that change would mean giving up something else that really matters to you—or something you can't identify keeps holding you back. Or maybe, even though you know you *want* to make a particular change, you don't believe you *can* make that change or you can't see a way to make it happen.

Although the issue might be a new one, it wouldn't be surprising if you'd been dealing with this dilemma for years, wrestling with indecision and inaction. That's because, when it comes to important life issues, *it's normal to get stuck*. And the variety of habits, situations, and patterns that people can get stuck in is staggering:

- Drinking, doing drugs, smoking, gambling, shopping, or having sex so much or so recklessly that you hurt your health, your career, your finances, or the people you care about.
- Struggling to gain control over your diet or your weight.
- Knowing you should exercise more but never managing to do it (or giving up each time you get started).
- Staying in a relationship, job, or career that you think you should leave.
- Losing control of your emotions and acting destructively or suppressing your emotions and feeling lost, empty, or frustrated.
- Holding on to resentment that you wish you could let go of or struggling to decide whether to forgive someone who's hurt you.
- Procrastinating about taking care of any number of tasks, small and large, all the while knowing you need to get moving.

Regardless of the issue and how long you've been grappling with it, you most likely picked up this book to see if it can help you get unstuck. I believe that it can. This book is based on the framework, strategies, and spirit of *motivational interviewing*, a counseling approach with a track record of effectiveness at helping people resolve even long-standing dilemmas about change in a remarkably short time.

Don't be thrown by the name. Motivational interviewing (or "MI," as it's known for short) has nothing to do with journalism or job interviews, and it's not a "rah-rah" method of motivating people. MI helps people who are thinking about a change to access their own natural, internal motivation and capacity for positive action. When offered by a counselor or healthcare provider, it's designed to be brief, and there's evidence from scientific studies that it can work in just a few sessions.[1] It can be the basis for a book as well because it works not primarily through the practitioner's knowledge or expertise but by recognizing and building on the fact that the most powerful force for change resides within you and that the key to helping you change is to help you find, strengthen, and act on it.

> Getting stuck in difficult life decisions is normal. Motivational interviewing provides an effective way of helping you resolve your own dilemma.

---

[1]If you're interested in the science behind motivational interviewing, an appendix describing this research and the history of the approach can be found at the end of the book.

The specifics of how MI can help you are found in the chapters to come. But it's possible to crystallize its essence in this simple way: Motivational interviewing will help you *listen to* yourself instead of *talking at* yourself and *understand* what's keeping you stuck instead of *demanding* of yourself that you get unstuck. As you give yourself "a good listening-to," with care and respect and without judgment, you will find yourself tapping into the natural well of internal motivation and ability for positive change that is present in all of us.

You might say, as one of the founders of MI has suggested, that participating in a motivational interview is like having a midwife present during childbirth. The midwife doesn't give birth to the baby; it's the mom who does all the hard work. But having someone who knows the ins and outs of helping the mom draw on her own strength and desire to give birth to a healthy child, who can guide her through a difficult yet life-changing process, can make all the difference. And that's what this book is designed to be: a step-by-step guide to capitalizing on the motivation and capacity for change that lies dormant within you, waiting to be born.

Now, people come to books like this with a variety of outlooks— hopeful and open-minded, skeptical, or just desperate for anything that might help. You'll soon be in a position to decide whether your initial attitude was justified and whether this book offers what you came looking for.

But first, I want to tell you about the one thing you *won't* find in this book. How you feel about what's missing will help you decide right now whether this book is right for you.

THE LAST THING YOU NEED IS ONE MORE PERSON TELLING YOU WHAT TO DO

This book will not tell you what to do about the issue in your life.

If you've been thinking about your issue long enough to pick up this book, then the chances are very good that at least one person has already been telling you what you should do and why. Whether the message came in the form of advice, persuasion, or a demand, the most important thing to notice is this: *here you are, still looking for help in getting unstuck.* People telling you what to do hasn't solved the problem. It may even have made the situation harder for you.

But isn't that strange? Granted, if someone seemed more interested in bossing you around than helping or was more critical than supportive, you probably didn't appreciate that at all. But if that person seemed to have your best interests at heart and knows you well or has lots of experience in dealing with issues like yours, why didn't this approach work?

Let's take a closer look. A person who knows you're struggling with some area of your life offers you advice about what to do. It's possible that you know right away that the advice won't work for you: you've tried it already, or it just doesn't feel like a good fit. (We'll come back to the key idea of "fit" in Part III of the book.) What do you do? You might say as much or you might smile politely, say "Thanks," and change the subject. Moreover, if the advice was really obvious—

- "Have you tried cutting out sweets?"
- "Maybe you should talk to your partner about it."
- "Remind yourself that you'll feel so much better once your work is out of the way."
- "What if you just limit yourself to drinking on social occasions and not by yourself?"

—your smile might be a bit forced as you wonder whether the person giving you the advice could really think you're so dense that you wouldn't have thought of that by now!

If the advice was *not* so obvious, and you haven't tried it before, you might just think, "Yeah, that's what I should do." And yet it doesn't really happen: maybe you try it a little bit and then give up; maybe time goes by and you forget or stop thinking about it until it gets brought up again, and you think, "Yeah, I should do that." From there, whether you just forget about it again, or start to feel bad about not taking the advice, the outcome is the same: nothing much changes.

Nothing, that is, except what happens the *next* time you see that person. If you think the subject will come up again, you might be tempted to avoid him or her. You don't really want to hear the same advice or hurt a well-meaning person's feelings by rejecting it.

And, of course, the person might do more than just ask how it's going or repeat the advice; he or she might start trying to *convince* you to follow it:

- "Don't you realize how good it would be for you to start exercising? You'd have so much more energy, you'd look better, and it's so good for your health!"
- "You really need to forgive your ex. It's just eating away at you, I can tell, and the only one it hurts is you."

- "You should start looking for a new job. Your boss doesn't appreciate you, and you're such a hard worker! I bet if you looked around, you'd find *ten* positions that are better than the one you have. Why don't you start sending around your resume and checking out the online job search sites?"

When you imagine someone saying something like this to you, can you start to feel the effect it has? The chances are pretty small that your reaction would be to think, "Of course! Why didn't I think of that? That's what I'll do!"

Instead, you might engage in *pseudoagreement*: "Oh, right, what a good idea, I'll do that," you'd say, smiling and nodding until you can change the subject or end the conversation. I call this the "bobblehead effect," and it's what people do every day when they visit their dentist and the hygienist asks how often they floss—they lie! Or, to put it more gently, they say what the hygienist wants to hear, fudge just a little, and smile and nod while the hygienist goes over the proper flossing technique yet again. This tactic is designed to avoid the lecture, minimize the embarrassment or guilt they're feeling about not flossing, or prevent the hygienist from thinking of them as "bad" or labelling them "noncompliant."

On the other hand, you might respond instead with a classic "yes, but . . ." statement:

- "I know it would be good for me to start exercising . . . but it's so hard to get started, and I have so little time."
- "I *should* forgive him, I really should; it would be so much better for me to just let go. . . . It's just that I can't get over how awful he acted. I just can't understand how he could have treated me that way."
- "You're right, I definitely deserve to be treated better at work—they'd be lost without me. . . . Still, things are really tough right now, and a lot of really good people are out there looking for positions—the competition would be so fierce."

These responses, you'll notice, leave you no closer to following the advice or making a change than you were when you started. In fact, instead of feeling more ready, willing, and able to take the steps being suggested, you're likely to feel even less so.

This is even more true when offers of advice or efforts at persuasion go one step further and turn into outright pressure. If you've ever been threatened with dire consequences if you don't do what someone says—

- "Either you quit drinking or I'm out of here!"
- "If you don't get your blood pressure under control right away, you're going to damage your kidneys and put yourself at serious risk of heart failure."

—or been the target of an effort to shame you—

- "How can you stay with him? Don't you have any self-respect?!"

—or make you feel so guilty that you'll be forced to change—

- "If you loved me, you'd take better care of your body instead of letting yourself go."
- "You're so selfish, spending all that money on clothes and other stuff you don't need, instead of saving it for things that are really important."

—then you know the effect of these kinds of tactics. Part of you might feel as though you must do what that person says, and you might even start thinking about how you're going to do it—and yet, at the exact same time, another part of you is having a very different reaction:

- Defiant: "You can threaten me all you want, but you can't make me!"
- Minimizing: "I know lots of people who do this much more than I do, and no one tries to tell *them* they have to stop."
- Anxious or panicky: "What am I going to do? I've got to do something! But what?!"
- Helpless and overwhelmed: "I know I have to stop . . . but I don't know how . . . this is awful."
- Consumed with guilt, shame, or self-loathing: "What's wrong with me? Why can't I act like a normal person?"

Unsolicited advice, rational persuasion, threats, or confrontation are all toxic to anyone who is stuck, trying fruitlessly to make or act on a decision. Unwanted efforts to direct your decisions or actions, no matter how well intended, only divert your energy and focus from wrestling with the problem to wrestling with the source of the pressure. They steer you toward avoiding, pretending, denying, or giving up. They leave you feeling deflated, demoralized, and generally worse about yourself than you already did.

And this brings us back to the reason for the statement I made at the beginning of this section: *This book will not tell you what to do about the issue in your life.*

Imagine that I'd begun by writing: *Stop hesitating and get started on changing your life! No more excuses; I know you can do it; it's time for you to get moving, and I'm going to show you how.* How would you have reacted? It's possible that in the moment you'd have felt relieved or even excited: "Yes! I'm going to do it now!" But it wouldn't have lasted; you'd have started to lose momentum; doubts would have crept in: "Do I really want to do this? Can I really carry it through? Is this really the right time?" And if you didn't feel this initial rush of enthusiasm, your reaction would almost certainly have been just like those I've been describing: superficial agreement plus minimizations or mental *yes buts*, indignation, guilt, shame, or helplessness at being unable to do what I was telling you to do.

HOW CAN THIS BOOK HELP?

The starting point for this book, and for MI as an approach to helping people with decisions about change, is this core insight: *There are good reasons you haven't yet decided about or made the change you've been considering.* When people are torn between competing wants and needs or visions of the future, they are in the state known as *ambivalence.* And ambivalence is seldom resolved through advice, persuasion, exhortation, confrontation, or coercion; all of those things tend to mire people even more deeply. So the way to free yourself to move forward is first to become interested in and accept the part of you that *doesn't* want to change—and to realize that this is a perfectly normal place to start the process.

The power of MI lies, in part, in its method for helping you reduce the pressure that has been building ever since you found yourself faced with a choice that you didn't feel ready, willing, or able to make. That pressure can come from outside, from others who become insistent or critical or impatient—but it also can, and often does, come from inside. In fact, as you'll see later, it's often because people have begun to put pressure *on themselves* that they react so strongly against the advice, persuasion, and direction of others.

Whether the pressure comes from inside, outside, or both, the more you feel pushed to "just do it," the more likely you are to struggle and feel trapped in a morass of indecision or to avoid dealing with the situation altogether. The good news is that the opposite is also true: once that pressure, both internal and external, is taken off, MI can guide you to find your own answers to the questions of what to do and how to do it.

THE WAY FORWARD

This book puts the power of motivational interviewing in your hands and offers concrete, practical steps for making and successfully carrying out whatever decision ultimately feels right for you. I'll begin by helping you understand why people get stuck when faced with difficult decisions about change and identify what's keeping *you* stuck. After introducing the critical dimensions of *importance* and *confidence* for change, I'll help you reduce the pressure you've been feeling and recognize and appreciate the positive qualities and strengths you already possess that can help you resolve your struggle. We'll explore your dilemma, tap into your most important values to turn them into the engines of positive change, and help you build confidence for tackling the challenges that lie ahead. When the time is right, I'll guide you in developing a personal plan for change that includes only the steps and strategies that feel right for you and then carrying out and sustaining the change you've undertaken.

Just as important as the content of this book (the "what") is the process I'll engage you in as you work your way through its chapters (the "how"). I'll invite you to write about your thoughts, feelings, and experiences related to the issue you're dealing with. To provide an easy way to keep your responses organized I've created online forms, with the same headings you'll find in this book, that are available for free at *www.guilford.com/zuckoff-forms*. (Of course, writing in a notebook or journal can work just as well if you prefer.)

As you answer questions that help you think in a fresh way about your dilemma, I'll often ask you to return to your answers and think (and write) more about them. This is what I meant by "giving yourself a good listening-to": a good listener does not just listen to the first thing you say, but keeps listening, inviting you to think further and deeper and discover things about yourself and your situation that you didn't realize before. (In fact, for reasons I'll explain later, I will at times quite literally ask you to "listen to yourself" as you read your responses out loud in order to help you think about them afresh.) Your understanding of your dilemma will change and grow as a result. This is how I'll help you find your own answers instead of giving you mine.

At every step along the way, what happens in this book will be guided by what the developers of MI, Drs. William R. ("Bill") Miller and Stephen

("Steve") Rollnick, have called the "spirit" of motivational interviewing. This spirit has four components:

1. *Acceptance,* which includes an abiding respect for the *autonomy* (*auto,* self; *nomos,* law: "to govern oneself") and affirmation of the worth of each person who is faced with a decision about change, as well as a desire to understand that person deeply and without judgment.

2. A commitment to *partnership,* the joining of the aspirations of the person facing the decision and the person who seeks to help that person achieve what he or she aspires to.

3. The belief that the most effective way of helping people succeed in making and carrying out their decisions is through *evocation,* or drawing out their own wishes, values, goals, strengths, and abilities, rather than attempts at installing "correct" ideas or expert information.

4. A strong sense of *compassion* for every person who struggles to make important life decisions without ever being certain that they are the right ones and to carry out those decisions in the face of obstacles and challenges that can easily derail change.

Wherever you are in dealing with the dilemma you're stuck in, that is the place where you will start. Because there is no single pathway through ambivalence, at times the activities you complete, and the order in which you complete them, will vary depending on what you need as you progress.

Similarly, there's no one "correct" pace at which to work with this book. Completing the activities in a particular section of a chapter together and finishing each chapter within a relatively short time can prevent you from losing your place. It's quite possible to complete all of Parts I and II within days or weeks, although Part III may take longer, depending (as you will see) on the kind of change you choose to make. What's most important, though, is to find the pace that feels right for you—not rushed or pressured, which would make it hard to remain thoughtful, but also not so slow or intermittent that you lose focus. Returning regularly to the activities in the book will give you the best chance of building momentum toward resolution of your dilemma.

Guided by the spirit of MI, and shaped by its research-proven methods, the book you are holding can be a source of support and a companion in your process of resolving your struggle with change. If you've decided this approach is right for you, let's get started.

You Don't Have to Change

1

Being Ambivalent

I have spoken to many groups of mental health, medical, addictions, and social work practitioners about how people change. Each time, I've asked those present to think of an area of their own lives in which they'd been considering whether or not to make a change and then to say how long they'd been considering it. With just a little prompting the majority of these therapists, counselors, doctors, nurses, caseworkers, and other professionals call out (sheepishly, forthrightly, or sometimes defiantly) "a few months," "a year," "2 years," "3 years," and then (to the increasing amusement and knowing nods of their colleagues) "5 years," "10," "20 . . . ."

When faced with important life decisions, it's *normal* for people to get stuck. This is as true for professional helpers as it is for you (and for everyone else, for that matter): they routinely, frustratingly, often exasperatedly get trapped in the all-too-human state known as ambivalence.

When one direction seems much preferable to another, most people have little trouble making a choice and pursuing the preferred option. But often the choice doesn't seem so clear. Ambivalence arises when people are confronted with a choice between two or more options, both (or all) of which are appealing or unappealing.

In some cases you are ambivalent when you're confronted with a choice between two things you really want—two good job offers or exciting relationship possibilities, say. In other cases, it's the opposite—you're unhappily forced to decide which is the lesser of two evils, like a person who's being blackmailed and has to choose whether to pay the blackmailer or have his secrets made public, or (to take an everyday example) a person who must decide between doing unpleasant chores or suffering the conse-quences of not doing them.

The most difficult kind of choice to make, though, is between two or more options, each of which has its good points and not-good points, or aspects that make you want to move toward it and aspects that make you want to move away.

The toughest choices to make are between options that each have pros and cons.

Simple examples or abstract descrip-tions of this kind of conflict can't do it jus-tice and won't help you work your way out of your own ambivalence. Instead, allow me to introduce five people who, like you, are caught in a dilemma. Their stories will bring home just how complex and sticky ambivalence can be and set the stage for a closer look at your own ambivalence—which will also be your first step toward understanding what it will take to resolve it.

MEET ALEC, BARBARA, COLIN, DANA, AND ELLIE

Alec: "People Want Me to Change, but I Don't Need To"

Alec is 39 years old and lives with his wife, Wendy, and 11-year-old daugh-ter, Jen, in the near suburbs of a small city. A salesman with a technology-based company, Alec is successful at his job, but it's a high-pressure posi-tion and he often feels stressed by it. He loves his family but doesn't get to spend as much time with them as he'd like to. He has a few friends but wouldn't say he's especially close with any of them. Most of the time Alec is either working or socializing with clients. Although he does have a hobby of gradually restoring an old muscle car (he bought it because it was the car he wanted as a kid), he doesn't seem to have much time to spend on this anymore either.

Alec is stuck in deciding what to do about his drinking. He would never identify himself as an alcoholic and would have choice words for anyone who described him that way. Most of the time he doesn't see his alcohol use as a problem at all—especially when others are trying to tell him that it *is* a problem. At those times he insists that he's a social drinker: part of his job is making connections with people in the companies he's trying to sell to, and getting together over a few drinks is the best way to make that happen. In fact, quitting drinking (as some people have been telling him he should do) would probably hurt his ability to do his job. He never misses work because of drinking, although he'll admit that on some days he might get off to a slow start after a late night entertaining clients.

He rarely gets drunk; most often he gets (as he puts it) "relaxed." And that seems like a good thing to him; he's always been kind of a high-strung guy who has a hard time sitting still, and drinking helps settle him down as well as acting as a great social lubricant.

As he sees it, Alec's biggest problem is that people in his life have been bugging him about his drinking recently, and he needs those people to believe that he takes what they're saying seriously so they'll back off. Wendy, his wife, is the main one. She's been giving him a hard time because he often comes home late after a few drinks, and when he finally does get home he's not in the mood to spend time with her or their daughter. She complains that she hardly sees him since either his evenings are taken up with client meetings or he's too tired after a few drinks for any quality time. She also thinks he's more likely to be irritable and start yelling after he's been drinking; he counters that he only gets mad because she just won't leave him alone to have some time to himself when he comes home, even though she knows he needs it and deserves it.

The other person who's been on his case lately, in Alec's view, is his primary care physician, who told Alec that he should cut down on his drinking because his cholesterol and blood pressure have been rising and he's put on some weight. While none of these issues are immediate threats, the doctor said, staying on this track would put Alec's health more at risk the older he gets. Alec got irritated with his doctor and dismissed the warnings, telling himself that he's still in great shape and doesn't need to start acting like an old man just yet. But a couple of weeks ago a friend at work, who is a few years older than Alec, and whom he respects as an excellent salesman and someone he can talk to about life and its hassles, told Alec about a scare he'd had recently—"not a heart attack, just some fibrillations"—and added that his doctor had told him he needed to stop drinking if he didn't want to have a much more serious event in the future. This got Alec thinking that he might want to cut down a little bit, kind of ease off for a while and maybe drop a few pounds too. He feels pretty sure that he could do that without much trouble, so he's started to think about it, even though a part of him doesn't want to give Wendy the satisfaction of saying "I told you so" or his doctor the idea that he thinks the warning was anything other than alarmist.

Barbara: "I Can't Go On Like This, I Must Go On Like This"

Barbara is 51 years old and lives with her husband of 30 years, Steve, in a gated community outside a large city. They have three children; the youngest, a daughter, just went off to college. Barbara met Steve in college; they got married at the end of her junior year (Steve had just graduated and gotten an entry-level position with a good company). She'd planned to go to law school after graduation but put it off when she got pregnant. When Steve's career began to take off, along with his income, she decided it was time to carry through with her plans and start law school. But when she became pregnant with their second child the demands became too great and she didn't go back to school for her third year.

Although she was disappointed not to have finished law school, Barbara happily threw herself into her life as a wife and mother. She became involved with all her children's activities—driving them to lessons after school, serving as an officer in the PTA, helping to coach her daughter's volleyball team and the robotics club after her older son showed an interest in it. She developed strong friendships with several of the mothers of her kids' friends and a wider circle of other women in the community. At the same time, as a result of her husband's often being away for work and her thorough involvement in her kids' lives, she and Steve had gradually drifted apart over the past two decades.

Barbara is stuck in thinking about ending her marriage. Steve is a good man and a good father; she feels fond of him and pictures them growing old together. She doesn't really want to leave him, and when she thinks about it she feels afraid of losing not only her financial security, but also the emotional security of knowing Steve cares and that she can count on him in a time of crisis. She also thinks about how ending the marriage would hurt him and also their children and how selfish it would be of her to tear apart their family; when she imagines it, her heart aches and she feels like a bad person.

And yet . . . in the empty house with Steve at work or traveling and her children gone she is acutely aware of how quickly time is passing and of how fast she is aging. She feels something in her life is missing and increasingly thinks this could be her last chance at developing a sense of passion about either a career or a relationship with a man—which she feels might be possible for her but which, she now admits to herself, she has never really experienced. In fact, she has recently had a mild flirtation with another man, a divorced father she'd known for a while through her daughter's volleyball team, who had complimented her on her outfit and asked if she'd like to have coffee sometime. She'd said no, but it scared her that she couldn't stop thinking about the encounter and wondering whether she should have said yes. When she's honest with herself, she realizes that she's afraid of life being the same forever, of missing out on opportunities for growth and excitement, and of growing old without ever knowing what it's like to experience them.

Barbara finds herself thinking about her situation almost constantly. Telling herself she must choose between her family and her own needs, she cannot accept having to give up either. When she talks to her sister, Sue, the only person she trusts enough to confide in, she feels intensely guilty, because her sister thinks Steve is such a good man. But her husband is also a conventional man, who seems happy with the state of their marriage and with knowing that she is there, at home, taking care of their life— and when she sees couples who are obviously in love, or reads about high-powered women in positions of authority, she feels a lump in her throat, wants to cry, and despairs that life is passing her by. Stymied every way she turns, she comes back again and again to the thought that no matter what she does it will be the wrong thing.

Colin: "Why Am I Still Acting This Way?"

Colin is 32 years old and has been in a stable relationship for the past 5 years with Paul, a man 12 years his senior. He has a good job in a creative field; it's a high-pressure position with long hours but he can't really imagine doing anything else. Paul has a high-level position in finance and works long hours as well. They have a dog but no children and have an upscale lifestyle, sharing a condo in a large and progressive city.

Colin is stuck in what to do about the way he expresses anger. Ever since adolescence his family and friends had known Colin as a person with a short temper. He knew they saw him this way, and at times he had wondered if his anger was too intense and even out of control, yet often Colin has felt as though people were exaggerating the problem. Yes, he might blow up sometimes, but most of the times this happened he believed he had good reason to be angry—someone had treated him disrespectfully, not shown the same consideration to him as he did to others, or failed him in some important way.

The main impetus for Colin's thinking about handling angry feelings differently is coming from his partner. From Paul's perspective, living with Colin is like riding a roller coaster. The highs can be very high: much of the time Colin is sweet, considerate, thoughtful, and affectionate. But the lows—when Colin, as he puts it, "explodes"—are very low. Paul tells Colin that often when Colin gets angry he feels blindsided, as if the anger comes out of nowhere. As a result, he says, he lives with a constant, low-level worry that at any moment Colin could go off on him. At times this has happened in public, and those episodes were especially painful for Paul: mortifying, as well as hurtful. But the cumulative effect of Colin's blow-ups, says Paul, has been to make him feel bad about himself. Worse, Paul has found himself taking these feelings out on others, angrily chastising his subordinates at work and even yelling at their dog for making messes.

When Paul describes what it's like to be the target of his anger, Colin feels sorry and regretful. Yet when he thinks about Paul's complaints, he also feels a certain amount of resentment. After all, he never gets physically violent; other than a few occasions when he might have pounded a table, and once when he threw a glass across the room, all he ever does is yell. Isn't that what people do when they get angry? he asks himself. Isn't that normal? He doesn't expect his partner to act any differently: Paul can yell at him, and does, just as he yells at Paul. And why won't Paul understand that what gets him really incensed is when Paul refuses to acknowledge that he has a right to be angry when he's been treated unfairly? If only Paul would validate my feelings, Colin thinks, so many of our worst arguments could have been avoided, or at least could have been settled much more quickly.

Despite this sense of justification, Colin has come to believe that he needs to do something to change the way he deals with angry feelings. He knows that he has become more frequently irritable and snappish with Paul, so the good times and warm feelings have been fewer and farther between. In fact, recently he's become aware of an increasing emotional distance between them; they seem to connect less often, and their sex life has become more intermittent. And after going for therapy, Paul told him that he doesn't want to live this way anymore—he loves Colin, but unless Colin's outbursts cease he doesn't think he can continue to be with him.

Because Paul said this in sorrow, rather than as an ultimatum, Colin did not feel threatened and doesn't feel like arguing back. He loves Paul, does not want to lose the relationship, and has decided to control himself and handle his anger differently. He believes it should not be too difficult since he knows when his anger is building and is sure he has the ability to restrain himself instead of just giving in to it. Yet he hasn't been very successful at controlling his anger thus far, and this has confused him and allowed some doubt to begin to creep in. He wonders what would happen if he *didn't* make this change and has become somewhat uncertain about how he's going to do what he needs to do to get himself under control.

Dana: "My Heart Says Yes, My Head Says No"

Dana is 26 years old and single, with no children. She lives alone in an apartment in a medium-size city. Dana was the first in person in her family to get a college degree, and after graduation she took a position as an administrative assistant with a large company. She was earning a good salary for someone with a BA early in her career and felt good about being able to establish her independence. Several of her friends from college, who went on to graduate school, told her how envious they were of her nice apartment and clothes and her ability to pick up the check when they went out for drinks. Her family has also been vocal about their pride in her and their gratitude that she has been able to help out her younger brother as well as several other family members financially. But recently, after almost 4 years on the job, Dana has been wondering about the choices she's made.

Dana is stuck in the decision of whether or not to leave her job and change careers. Her job is steady and reliable, the company stable, the salary sufficient (with regular raises), the responsibilities manageable and familiar. Yet for some time now she's been feeling restless and dissatisfied. Two of her bosses tend to talk down to her and treat her as less capable than she really is, and she's not getting the opportunities for advancement she'd hoped for. She's begun to find her daily routine boring, and the good feelings that come from knowing she's taking care of her family have begun to be outweighed by feeling bad about the lack of respect she receives. Her friends, having finished graduate school and begun working in their fields, are not only catching up to her financially but, as their careers as professionals have begun to take off, their conversation is mostly about their excitement about the work they are doing.

Dana feels drawn to teaching, and knowing that her friends are pursuing their dreams has left her thinking more and more about what it would be like to pursue her own. She's always loved taking care of children, and her own experience of succeeding in school in challenging circumstances as a result of her parents' encouragement and the attention of a few special teachers makes her want to pass these gifts along. When she thinks about going back to school for her master's degree in education, she gets excited. Yet at the same time she tells herself she could never do anything like that. She worries a bit about the academic demands—she'd been out of the loop for a while; would graduate school be more than she can handle? But what feels like the main obstacle is that her financial situation would get worse for her before it got better.

When Dana mentions her idea to her family, they tell her that she'd be foolish to give up her job to go back to school for a degree that would leave her earning less money than she does now with no great prospects for the future. As a grad student she wouldn't be able to support herself, they say; she could end up with loans she wouldn't be able to pay back and might even lose her apartment and end up homeless. Dana thinks their fears are exaggerated, and yet she knows she has no safety net; no one in her family is in a position to come to her rescue if things take a turn for the worse. She also feels guilty when she imagines leaving her job, knowing she would no longer be able to help her family financially, at least for a while. Still, she finds herself perusing career-search websites or looking at graduate school programs online while she's at work. When she lets herself imagine actually finding out more about these programs, she's flooded with anxiety, and as the panic rises she dismisses the thoughts as pipe dreams. But she can't let them go, so she continues to surf the Web and think about what it would be like to just quit her job and do it.

Ellie: "Wise Up and Give Up?"

Ellie is 43 years old and lives with her husband, Gil, and their four children, ages 21, 15, 9, and 6, in a small town where she works as a counselor at a community mental health agency and Gil works as shipping foreman in a manufacturing company. Ellie and Gil were high school sweethearts. After graduation he was hired for a low-skill job by the company he's still with and worked his way up into a position of responsibility. She went to a community college and then had a series of jobs before she found her current position, which she's held for 14 years, in which she helps people with mental illness develop the skills to live independently. Ellie finds her job frustrating at times and wishes it paid better, but it makes her feel good to know that she makes a difference in the lives of people worse off than she is.

Ellie is stuck in a long-term struggle with her weight. She desperately wants to be thinner and has been trying to make that happen off and on for most of her adult life. Most of the weight she wants to lose she gained during her pregnancies. After the birth of her first child, she worked hard and got back to her prepregnancy weight; it was still a little higher than her ideal but she was proud of herself nonetheless. However, with each of her following pregnancies she lost less weight than she had gained, feeling unhappy with herself all the while. Worse yet, since her youngest was born she'd been slowly but steadily gaining more, so that now she is about 45 pounds over the weight she wants to be.

Ellie feels upset and self-conscious about her weight most of the time, although she's learned to make jokes about it with her friends at work and pretend it doesn't bother her. In fact, she feels as though she thinks about her weight almost constantly, to the point where she gets so frustrated that she wants to scream. She has joined Weight Watchers and Overeaters Anonymous, bought books on weight loss and tried all kinds of diets, and tried various types of exercise she learned about from friends, magazines, the Internet, and even infomercials, but has always ended up back where she started or even worse off. Each time she's begun a diet or an exercise program she started enthusiastically and made progress—sometimes a little, sometimes a lot—but then couldn't seem to stick to either one in the face of various life challenges that popped up. Quitting has made her feel deflated, self-critical, and hopeless, and these feelings have made her want to eat even more.

Ellie's life is busy and stressful; she feels as though she has very little time for herself and is always on the go. She loves her husband, and he loves her, but he works long hours and is exhausted when he comes home, so he's not around much to help with household chores or even to just spend time together. She is solely responsible for taking care of the children and for cooking for the family. Gil likes meat and potatoes, and her children all like different things (her 15-year-old has recently declared herself a vegetarian), and she finds herself spending a couple of hours every night after she gets home from work in the kitchen preparing meals, where she ends up snacking and never getting around to sitting down to her own meal until late in the evening.

Eating is something Ellie does to keep her energy up and to have a little pleasure; she eats comfort foods at home and snacks at work, and if anyone comments (as her well-meaning girlfriends have been known to do), she replies that on some days, sitting down to eat for a few minutes is the only break she gets. Her husband has learned not to comment about her eating or her weight, and he feels bad because he knows how much she struggles with it. Trying to be reassuring, he says he loves her no matter how she looks, but when she hears him say such things she feels more despairing than ever, knowing he doesn't really understand what it's like for her. Lately, she finds herself thinking she should just learn to live with herself the way she is, so at least she could stop feeling like a failure all the time.

FIVE KINDS OF AMBIVALENCE, ONE HUMAN DILEMMA

Ambivalence comes in many varieties and flavors, all unpleasant. Each of the five people you've met is ambivalent about an issue in his or her life, yet each is stuck in a different way and for different reasons.

- Alec feels that the conflict is mostly between him and the people in his life who want him to change; he has a vague inkling that he might need to change but a stronger sense that the people around him are wrong, unreasonable, unfair, and don't understand him. When he considers his drinking, Alec is much more aware of how it helps him deal with his life than he is of any negative consequences that it's begun to bring about.
- Barbara, dissatisfied in her marriage, feels torn between putting her own wishes first, or even treating them as if they matter, and

taking care of those she loves. Or rather, that's the conflict she's focused on; the tension between her own competing needs and desires (security and comfort vs. passion and fulfillment) is not so clear to her. Nonetheless, Barbara believes that choosing one way or the other would require her to give up something that matters, and not knowing whether she can accept the inevitable loss, she is consumed with ruminating about which one she should choose.

• Like Alec, Colin is being prompted to consider a change by his partner's complaints. However, Colin views the effects of his behavior on the person he loves with concern, and as his responsibility to address, so he is perplexed that thus far he's been unable to change it. The possibility that his own mixed feelings about how he expresses anger might have something to do with this incapacity has not yet occurred to him.

• Dana, like Barbara, is dissatisfied with the way things are going in her life. But unlike Barbara, who feels thoroughly torn between two compelling possibilities, Dana knows in her heart what she really wants to do. Yet her fear of the consequences of taking that step, risking what she has for what she wants, keeps her from acting; her mistrust of her own judgment ("Am I really making the right decision?") is leaving her hanging, on the precipice, hesitant and unable to move forward.

• Ellie, too, knows what she wants to change and in fact has long been trying to change it. However, she no longer believes she can succeed. Her confidence has been undermined, so she vacillates between being ready to take action and the sinking feeling that to do so is pointless, a waste of her limited energy, and a kind of self-cruelty in getting her own hopes up only to see them dashed. Because Ellie has not made any connection between the state of her life and her struggle to lose weight, she blames herself for her failures and in turn feels more and more helpless to make changes she wants.

Your ambivalence, like the ambivalence of these five people, may take one of a number of forms: staying the same and making a change may each seem desirable; staying the same and making a change may each seem *un*desirable; every option may have both desirable and undesirable aspects; you may know that you want to change but believe it's not possible, or fear the unfamiliar, or worry about others' reactions.

Yet as different as the problems, circumstances, and sources of "stuckness" experienced by these five people are, there are also several common threads that highlight aspects of ambivalence that you will need to be aware of to find your own way through it.

One is that *the decisions about the people, issues, and areas of our life that are most important to us are the ones we are most likely to get stuck in.* The more a decision matters, the more closely we look at all the advantages and disadvantages of each possible option. As a result, we are that much more aware of all the reasons both to choose and not to choose each possible pathway, and it's easy for us to become buried in the details and lost in the complexity of the decision we're facing. So *one key to resolving ambivalence is to find a way to untangle all the complicated and conflicting thoughts we have about the issue we're struggling with so that we can restore our ability to think our way through it.*

At the same time, because getting the decision right is so important to us, *we're much less willing to go with what seems the slightly better option than if we were confronting a minor issue.* When choosing between two flavors of ice cream we may like one only a little bit better than another—but that little bit is enough to tip the balance. When choosing between staying at a reliable but boring job and giving up financial stability to go back to school for a career we might love or between a familiar, well-loved source of pleasure and well-being that's also hurting us and an uncertain and unfamiliar alternative, we're not willing to settle for "slightly better"—we want to feel as though the direction we're choosing is definitely the right one. Yet the desirability of the pathways before us may seem so similar—and worse, might look much more like a comparison, not even of apples and oranges, but of apples and light bulbs (that is, two completely different kinds of things)—that we just don't feel willing to give up one for the other.

It is the nature of being human, of course, that we must make our choices despite our inability to know with certainty ahead of time that the choice we make will bring us the results we hope for. Yet when the stakes are this high, we're very reluctant to settle for "maybe"; we want to feel certain and for the choice to be clear. So *a second key to resolving ambivalence is to find a way of achieving a feeling of being settled or at peace with the decision we have made.*

A third commonality among all kinds of ambivalences is that *the more a decision matters to us, the more emotionally triggered we become when considering it.* When it comes to important life decisions, we don't just evaluate the situation dispassionately; our feelings become involved. Ambivalence, then, is a complex cognitive–affective state.[1] Rationally, our reasons to do

---

[1]Leffingwell, T. R., Neumann, C. A., Babitzke, A. C., Leedy, M. J., & Walters, S. T. (2007). Social psychology and motivational interviewing: A review of relevant principles and recommendations. *Behavioural and Cognitive Psychotherapy*, *35*, 31–45.

one thing conflict with reasons not to or to do something else; emotionally, we may experience excitement at the possibility of life getting better, fear that life will get worse, worry about whether we're seeing things clearly or making a mistake, hope for the future, guilt at the prospect of hurting someone we care about, or sadness about whatever we will have to give up.

Experiencing emotions as we wrestle with a decision about change is not just inevitable but also valuable. Feelings are our guides to what we want and what we care about, as well as to the meanings of others' behavior toward us. Anger tells us that we're being treated unfairly, for example; sadness that we are losing something important to us; shame that we are being judged inadequate. Without our feelings we'd be as lost as Data on *Star Trek: The Next Generation* or Sheldon Cooper on *The Big Bang Theory*. The trouble is that high levels of emotion interfere with our ability to think clearly about what we want, to weigh our options and come to a decision that *feels* right to us. Even if intellectually one choice seems better than another, the emotions we're experiencing can make it hard to arrive at that good sense of certainty and security that we instinctively look for to tell us that we've made the right decision. So *a third key to resolving ambivalence is to find a way to allow our feelings to inform our decision making without overwhelming and derailing it.*

This brings us to the final commonality among all forms of ambivalence. Lost in the complexity of the choice we're facing, struggling to determine whether any of our options is the one that will take us where we want to go, and flooded with feelings that can cloud our judgment, our tendency is to get entangled in unproductive arguments with ourselves. Soon there are two (or more) conflicting voices in our head, arguing one way and then another:

"You've really got to make a decision."

"I know, but what am I going to do? "

"You might as well just take a chance and do something. How bad could it be?"

"Pretty bad! It could all go wrong. How am I supposed to deal with all the stress?"

"Well then, just forget about it. Live with things the way they are."

"But things are not good the way they are. I want them to be better."

"Then do something about it!"

"But what?"

Like a cartoon character pacing back and forth, wearing a groove in the ground so deep that all the character can see is the path ahead and the path behind, a person stuck in ambivalence can soon feel trapped in point-lessly retracing his or her mental steps, repeating the same arguments again and again, and never getting anywhere except more mired in indecision. It can become almost impossible to think outside those familiar mental pathways, which can begin to seem like the only way to think about the problem or situation, and soon convince the ambivalent person that there's no solution, no way out. And this rumination, in turn, leads to *the terrible triad of ambivalence*, the most stubborn and potent contributors to getting and staying stuck: *anxiety, avoidance, and self-blame.*

People are not made to tolerate the back-and-forth, frustrating, cognitively and emotionally overwhelming state of ambivalence. As we wrestle with an important life decision we grow increasingly *anxious*, that unpleasant feeling that tells us that we're at risk of something bad happening to us without knowing what that something is. Unsurprisingly, the more anxious we become, the more motivated we are to look for some way to reduce the feeling. If we could resolve the conflict, our anxiety would naturally disappear. But what happens when we can't resolve the conflict, no matter how hard we try?

Every instinct tells us that when our efforts are futile, the smartest thing to do is to stop trying—turn our attention to or invest our energy in something else that's likely to benefit us. And in many situations this instinct serves us well; unable to succeed at one goal, we accept reality and find another to pursue. Unfortunately, when we get stuck in ambivalence it is precisely because we can neither succeed at making a decision nor live with being undecided. So when we turn away from the conflict in which we're stuck, we're not moving on—we're bringing ourselves temporary relief from anxiety by avoiding it. And sometime soon—whether hours, days, weeks, or even months later—we are going to find ourselves, since nothing has been resolved, back in the same exact spot we were in before:

"Now you've *really* got to make a decision."	"I know, but what am I going to do?"
"You can't keep doing this. Do something! Take a chance!"	"But I can't! What if things go wrong?"
"Well then, forget about it. Live with things the way they are."	"But I don't want to. There has to be a way to make this better."
"Then do something about it!"	"I know! I want to. But what?"

Take a moment and notice how you feel after reading these statements. Annoyed? Impatient? Now think about this: when stuck in ambivalence, people repeat these internal dialogues dozens or even hundreds of times over weeks, months, or years. Talk about frustration! With no new information to add to our decision process—since we have, after all, been avoiding thinking about the situation since the last time we tried to figure it out—the "conversations" in our heads get repeated almost verbatim, generating a sense of futility that only intensifies the miserable cycle of anxiety-provoking mental conflict alternating with avoidance.

And this feeling of futility brings on self-blame. Angry and frustrated at being unable to get unstuck, we turn on ourselves, certain that there must be a solution that we're just not seeing or that anyone else would have dealt with this situation long ago. We tell ourselves that we're weak, lazy, or stupid, that something must be wrong with us to be going around and around in circles and getting nowhere. Sometimes we do this as a form of "tough love": if we're only hard enough on ourselves, we think, we'll finally do what's difficult and move on with our lives. Sometimes we do this for no purpose at all, but just because we feel like failures or that we deserve to feel bad. Either way, the combination of anxious avoidance and

- -

Four Keys to Resolving Ambivalence

1. **The decisions that are most important to us are the ones we are most likely to get stuck in . . .** . . . so one key to resolving ambivalence is to find a way to untangle all the complicated and conflicting thoughts we have about the issue we're struggling with so we can restore our ability to think our way through it.

2. **When a decision is important, we're much less willing to accept the slightly better option . . .** . . . so a second key to resolving ambivalence is to find a way of achieving a feeling of being settled or at peace with the decision we have made.

3. **The more a decision matters to us, the more emotionally triggered we become when considering it . . .** . . . so a third key to resolving ambivalence is to find a way to allow our feelings to inform our decision-making without overwhelming and derailing it.

4. **Falling into circular, unproductive arguments with ourselves triggers the terrible triad of ambivalence . . .** . . . so a fourth key to resolving ambivalence is to break the cycle of internal argumentation, anxiety, avoidance, and self-blame.

- -

self-blame—which go together, of course: the worse thinking about our situation makes us feel, the more we try to avoid thinking about it; the more we avoid thinking about it, the more we stay stuck and the worse we feel about ourselves and our situation—drives us ever deeper into the very state that provoked them. So *a fourth key to resolving ambivalence is to break that cycle of internal argumentation, anxiety, avoidance, and self-blame.*

THE STORY OF YOUR AMBIVALENCE

Now that we've taken a closer look at what it's like to be stuck in ambivalence, and you've read the stories of five ambivalent people, it's time for you to describe your own issue. (You'll find an online form for this activity, titled "The Story of My Ambivalence," at *www.guilford.com/zuckoff-forms*, or you can write in your journal.) It's important to write about your situation thoughtfully and in detail. This does not mean you should expect to figure out what to do or which direction to head in as you write about it! Your goal here is not to solve the problem. If you could do that now you'd already have done it—and all that's likely to happen if you try is that you will tread one more time the same circular, frustrating, self-blaming mental pathways. Also—and this is very important—don't expect yourself to be consistent in what you write. If it all made sense, you wouldn't be stuck! It's a hallmark of ambivalence that people contradict themselves; don't try to censor contradictions or make everything fit together neatly and coherently.

Instead, focus on simply describing the issue you are struggling with in light of what you've read and thought about so far. As you're writing, think about the following questions as prompts to help you capture as fully as possible the thoughts and feelings you have about the situation you are in:

- Describe the history of the issue you're ambivalent about. How long have you been dealing with it? What have you previously tried to do to make a decision, solve the problem, or achieve some form of change? How have your thoughts, feelings, wishes, and fears related to the issue changed over time?

- The mixed feelings and conflicting thoughts of ambivalence often take the form of two (or more) sides of an argument, or "voices" expressing different views or wishes about what to do or what the right choice is. What's the argument you've been having with yourself? What are these different voices saying now? What have you been telling yourself recently about what you want and don't want, hope for and fear, should do and shouldn't do?

- Who are the people involved in or affected by the issue? What have they been telling you about what they want you to do or what they think the best decision is? How do you feel about what each of these people has been saying to you or about what you believe they think you ought to do?

IMPORTANCE AND CONFIDENCE: KEY DIMENSIONS OF MOTIVATION

Getting unstuck and moving from ambivalence to *resolution* (knowing what you intend to do and committing to doing it) and *action* (doing what you've committed to do) is a step-by-step process. The first step is to recognize that what people usually think of as *being motivated* has two dimensions: *importance* and *confidence*.

Importance

Naturally, people become increasingly motivated to change when they begin to view their current behavior, situation, or pattern as a problem for them. (Notice that this is not the same as someone else thinking you have a problem; importance increases only if you come to share this perception or feel concerned about how the other person sees your behavior.)

But perceiving a problem isn't enough. People see problems all the time without being able to decide what to do about them—that's another way of describing ambivalence. For importance to increase enough to resolve ambivalence, you have to see the *benefits* of pursuing a path as clearly and dramatically outweighing the *costs* of doing so. And the truth is, when it comes to important life decisions, just about every option a person is faced with has costs as well as benefits, no matter how clear the benefits are. Sure, losing weight and getting into shape will improve your health, give you more energy and zest, enhance your self-esteem, and maybe even make you more popular—but it may also require you to give up sleep to work out in the morning, or lose time with family in the evenings, give up some of your favorite foods, or tolerate feeling hungry instead of satisfied. . . . It's only when the advantages of going in one direction seem much greater than its disadvantages (which is also to say that the advantages of one option are clearly superior to the advantages of others) that the balance tips.

But then, what do I mean by "dramatically outweighs"? How superior is "clearly superior"? To really understand how the "importance" dimension of ambivalence gets resolved, we have to go beyond "costs and benefits" in the everyday sense and recognize that ultimately how important making a change (or not making a change) is to you has to do with your *values*.

Here's an illustration: Imagine that I told you there existed a special pill that, if taken once a day at the same time, would cause you to live to be 100 and never be sick a day in your life. Would you take it? Of course—the benefits of the pill far outweigh the minor inconvenience. But now imagine that I told you that to receive the pill you would have to agree never to see any of the people you love again. Would you agree to this bargain?

> People become ready to change when the benefits clearly outweigh the costs . . . and it's our values that tip the balance.

A long, healthy life is something that almost anyone would want, and most people would be willing to make sacrifices to have it. But most of us value the people we love in our life even more than we value our health— and when competing options provoke a conflict of values, you will almost always choose the option that matters to you most, even if it does bring costs of its own.

Confidence

Imagine another scenario: A person decides that doing something would bring many benefits and few costs and that choosing this option is not just completely consistent with her values but would help her live out those values more fully. Can we anticipate with certainty that she will make that choice?

The answer is no. What she does will depend not only on how important the goal is but also on whether she believes she can get there. If she expects her efforts to be fruitless, to fail time and again, the chances are very good that she will not even bother to try. And after all, why should she? What would be the point of banging her head against the wall if all she's going to end up with is a splitting headache?

Resolution of ambivalence involves not only knowing the path that is right for you but also feeling confident about pursuing it—believing you can succeed at accomplishing what you hope to accomplish. In contrast, when a person believes she has a problem, but also believes there's nothing she can do to solve it, she really has only two options: denial or despair. That is, she can tell herself that she really *doesn't* have a problem (or that it's not so bad), or she can face the idea that the problem is really serious but completely unsolvable and become consumed by hopelessness. Obviously, neither of these possibilities is a good one, which highlights how crucial confidence is in the process of getting unstuck.

What influences how confident a person feels about succeeding at something? The most powerful factor is our previous experience of success and failure: successes build confidence and failures erode it, unless we decide the failure was just a setback and we'll be able to succeed if we try a different approach. But it's not just our history with a particular pursuit that shapes our beliefs about what we can accomplish; perceived successes in one area that's important to us build our confidence that we can succeed in others, just as perceived failures in important areas can dent our confidence in general. And most broadly, how we feel about ourselves overall—our general self-evaluation or self-esteem—can also play a role in whether we feel able to tackle any given challenge that we face.

> People become ready to change when they believe they can succeed . . . and it's our successes and failures, and how they've made us feel about ourselves, that shape those beliefs.

RATING IMPORTANCE AND CONFIDENCE

If importance and confidence are the key factors for resolving ambivalence and strengthening motivation and commitment to action, then increasing them should be our ultimate focus, and identifying whether one dimension of motivation or the other is really holding you back is our next step. It could be that a given option is highly important to you, yet your confidence for carrying it out is low; on the other hand, your confidence that you can succeed may be high enough that you'd be moving ahead if only you felt sure which direction is right for you. Or it might be that you're both unsure about what you should do and doubtful that you could do it even if you were sure.

So the next thing I'm going to ask you to do is to rate the importance of making the change you're considering and your confidence about doing so. First, though, I'm going to share with you how each of the five ambivalent people you met earlier in this chapter rated themselves on these dimensions and their comments on why they gave themselves the ratings they did.

Importance and Confidence

How **important** is it to me *right now* to make the change I am considering?

0	1	2	3	4	5	6	7	8	9	10

Not at all   Moderately   Extremely

How **confident** am I *right now* that I would be able to make that change?

0	1	2	3	4	5	6	7	8	9	10

Not at all   Moderately   Extremely

Alec: Low Importance, High Confidence

Alec, whose issue is his drinking, gives himself a **3** for importance and a **9** for confidence:

> "I could cut back if I wanted to, and maybe I will. But things are going well for me at work, and if I really had an alcohol problem, do you think I'd be able to say that? I love my wife, but her whole family thinks that anyone who has a couple of drinks is an alcoholic. And my doctor, well, I think he was out of line trying to tell me what I should do; he doesn't know anything about my life, and I've never felt healthier. Believe me, if my drinking got to be a problem, I'd take care of it. That's the kind of guy I am; I do what needs to be done. Look, I know everybody means well. And maybe it wouldn't hurt my waistline to ease off a bit. But everyone needs to take a step back and let me handle my own life."

Barbara: Moderate Importance, Low Confidence

Barbara, who is wrestling with whether or not to leave her husband, gives herself a **5** for importance and a **2** for confidence:

> "I just don't know what the right thing to do is, and I feel so helpless. There's so much more I want from life, and so much more I'm capable of. Sometimes I feel as though time is running out, and I can't let myself waste another day waiting, I have to leave. But then as soon as I have that thought, all I can think about is how hurt my husband would be and how much it would upset the kids, and also, if I'm honest, how scary it would be for me to be on my own after all these years.

So I just feel torn and trapped, and there's nothing I can do. And no matter what I decide, someone is going to pay an enormous price."

Colin: High Importance, Moderately High Confidence

Colin, who is having trouble with how he expresses anger, gives himself an 8 for importance and a 7 for confidence:

> "Even though I think a lot of the things I get angry about would make anyone mad, I know I need to do something about my temper. Paul is very sensitive, and my explosions have had a negative effect on him and our relationship. I feel upset about that. I want us to be happy together like we were at the beginning. I know I can get this under control if I put my mind to it. I think I haven't really done that yet, and that must be why I keep having those bad moments. I guess I have to get serious, because I don't want to lose him."

Dana: Moderate Importance, Moderately Low Confidence

Dana, who is trying to decide whether to leave her job to go back to school and pursue a different career, gives herself a 6 for importance and a 4 for confidence:

> "I'm pretty sure I'd be happier as a teacher than I am as an administrative assistant, but the situation is more complicated than that. People count on me, so I can't just do whatever I feel like doing. Besides, I like being able to take care of myself, and it would feel like going backward to become a student again and have to ask for help instead of giving it. Still, I have to admit that the idea of spending the rest of my life doing this type of work is pretty grim, even if I was able to work my way up into a position with more responsibility. I'm good with children, and I know I could make a difference as a teacher. I just don't see how I could get there from here."

Ellie: Very High Importance, Very Low Confidence

Ellie, who wants to lose weight, gives herself a 10 for importance and a 0 for confidence:

> "I am so tired of this battle. I've wanted to lose weight for a million years, and I just can't do it. I've tried everything, and nothing works.

I remember how good I felt about myself when I was thin—not too thin, you know, just in good shape. Even though I'm older now, I know I could still look and feel a lot better, too, if I could get this darn weight off me. But with my kids and my job and my husband, there just isn't enough time in the day to take care of myself, and maybe I should just accept that I can't lose weight and stop driving myself crazy."

Assessing Importance and Confidence: Your Turn

Now it's time for you to rate your own level importance and confidence for change. Please go back and reread what you wrote about your ambivalence. (As I noted earlier, creating a cycle of writing, rereading, reflecting, and writing again will be one of the most important ways to help you move through and resolve it.)

Next, choose the number that best captures your feelings about the importance of making the change you've been considering and your confidence that you could succeed at making that change if you decided to do it, circling the numbers under the questions on page 31 or using the form at *www.guilford.com/zuckoff-forms*. Once you've done so, please describe why you chose the numbers you did in your journal or the online form.

Your Ambivalence and Theirs

In thinking about what you've written in response to the activities in this chapter, you might have noticed similarities between your ambivalence or your levels of importance and confidence and those of Alec, Barbara, Colin, Dana, or Ellie. You may also have found that the thoughts, feelings, or situation of one of them resonated especially strongly with you. If so, I'd like you to look at those reactions more closely. Please ask yourself the following questions and write down your answers (either in your journal or in the online form titled "My Ambivalence and Theirs" at *www.guilford.com/zuckoff-forms*):

- In what ways do you identify with that person?
- What might you be able to learn so far from the story of his or her ambivalence or his or her responses to the importance and confidence questions?
- How is your situation unique?

The five ambivalent people you've read about in this chapter will accompany you throughout this book. Each time I ask you to respond to questions or complete an activity I will invite you to consider their responses before you formulate your own.

Following the progress of all five companions as they work alongside you to complete the book's activities may help you think more clearly about your own dilemma and give you a variety of illustrations and perspectives to consider. However, if you find all five stories more than you can keep track of, you might prefer to focus primarily on the one person you relate to most strongly or whose ambivalence most closely resembles your own. Or you might want to find a middle ground: reading all the responses when you're less sure how to respond to an activity but being more selective when you know how you want to respond right away. If you read some of the responses and then realize you're not making as much progress as you'd hoped, you might decide to go back and read all the responses more thoroughly. What matters most is that you find the way to adapt the companions' stories, struggles, and successes that best support your own efforts to get unstuck and move ahead.

RESOLVING YOUR AMBIVALENCE: WHERE YOU'RE STARTING FROM

By identifying your importance and confidence for change, you have begun to clarify what has been keeping you from resolving your ambivalence. People make decisions and take action when both importance and confidence for change are high. You are not feeling stuck because you're weak, lazy, or foolish; you're stuck because you have not been at a level of importance, confidence, or both that would allow you to move forward.

Helping you develop a sense of resolution about the direction ahead and a belief in your ability to get there will be our goal. Remarkably, you can begin to increase both of these dimensions of motivation by *removing* rather than *adding* something. The next two chapters will explain what I mean by this and show you how. But it all starts with this simple idea: *You don't have to change.*

2

The Pressure Paradox

"You don't have to change": it's literally and self-evidently true. People can spend years (even decades!) thinking about what they should or could or want to do, or taking one step forward and one step back, and never reach a final resolution. The nagging uncertainty and tension can sap the pleasure from life, but it is not fatal (even if the long-term effects of some kinds of behavior can be). So people can remain in this kind of limbo indefinitely and even change that's "necessary" may not happen.

But when someone says "You *have to* change," it's not really a statement of fact; it's meant as a plea, a warning, or most often a demand. And this is the message I wish to counter.

Regardless of what others insist you do, or what you might try to force yourself to do, no one can "make" you change, come to a final decision, or solve a problem you're facing. In fact, I would go even further: It's better *not* to make a decision or take action to change before you know where you want to go *and* believe you can get there.

Pressure to change usually has the *opposite* of the intended effect—it deepens stuckness rather than freeing you from it. This is the pressure paradox, and this chapter is devoted to helping you understand why it happens and how it interferes with your efforts to make progress on the dilemma you are struggling with.

AMBIVALENCE UNDER PRESSURE

In the abstract most people are apt to acknowledge that it's not possible to make another person change. You might know the old joke:

"How many therapists does it take to change a light bulb?"
"Only one, but the light bulb has to want to change."

Yet the belief that we can make people take action in their own interest persists in almost all of us, because it's terribly hard to accept that there's nothing we can do to stop the people closest to us from acting in ways that are harmful to themselves or to others. So family and friends nag, plead, or demand—yet their loved ones usually go on doing what they've been doing, whether what "has to" change is alcohol or drug use, chronic procrastination, an abusive relationship, or something else. Doctors and counselors, spouses and parents, employers and the legal system issue dire warnings or ultimatums—yet people on the receiving end often continue the same health or school or job or social behavior regardless of the suffering it may cause.

The frustration and helplessness people feel when their efforts to pressure someone to change fail can lead them to conclude that the person who refuses to do what seems obviously healthy or wise is *in denial.* Yet those who resist pressure to change are often, as I've been saying all along, quite well aware of and affected by the negative consequences of their situation. They are not "in denial" but stuck in ambivalence—and no amount of pressure will make ambivalent people become unstuck.

And this is not only true when pressure comes from others. While we typically acknowledge that we can't make other people change if they don't want to, we're much more likely to believe that it *is* possible to overcome our own hesitation about change by force—by mentally pressuring ourselves. But when we do this *we are treating ourselves the same way that others who want us to change treat us.* It's like we're split in two—one who suspects that something needs to change but isn't sure what that is, or what will happen as result, or how to do it; and one who, tense and miserable or impatient and angry or scornful or scared, tries to nag, plead, threaten, shame, or otherwise "make" himself or herself "just get on with it." Just for this reason, pressure from *inside* is no more likely to be effective in getting us to make decisions and move ahead before we are ready than pressure that comes from outside us.

Why do we recognize that we can't change others by force yet believe we can force ourselves to change?

WHY DOES PRESSURE BACKFIRE?

Defending Our Positive View of Ourselves: *"Don't Judge Me!"*

All of us are highly motivated to maintain positive feelings about ourselves. Call it self-esteem, self-regard, or self-enhancement—there is a universal human need to see ourselves as good, sensible, worthwhile people, and we devote a great deal of mental and emotional energy to making sure we do.

Pressure to change, though, conveys a different message: "There is something wrong with you. You're no good the way you are." This kind of negative judgment threatens our sense of worth. And *as with any other threat, we respond by trying to defend ourselves,* by insisting that we are not wrong, that our choices are not bad or mistaken, and that our behavior is perfectly acceptable and nothing to feel ashamed of. Think about the most recent time someone criticized you for something you did and insisted you should have done it differently. Do you recall your inner reaction, not necessarily what you said out loud but how you felt and what you wanted to say? Did it involve wanting to explain, justify, or otherwise defend what you had done?

Criticisms, put-downs, and blame can be even more powerful threats when they come from inside us rather than from other people. Negative judgments about ourselves are harder to escape and harder to argue against. We tend to believe our judgments of ourselves, and if we eventually become convinced that our negative self-judgments are correct, we may even seek out others who will confirm them, our need to believe that our view of ourselves is right outweighing even our need to view ourselves positively. Although we may fight the temptation to believe the negative things we think about ourselves, we can easily fall into a vicious cycle of plummeting self-regard, denying the negative messages ever more strenuously even as we sickeningly suspect that we really are foolish, worthless, or bad. Which, in turn, works against actually feeling ready, willing, or able to undertake positive changes by triggering an even stronger defense of how we already are.

> Our need to believe that we are our own best judges can overpower our need to feel good about ourselves.

Defending Our Autonomy: *"Don't Try to Control Me!"*

All of us are also highly motivated to feel in control of our own actions and decisions. Although the need for autonomy is often confused with a desire to be left alone, most people want relationships that are close *and* autonomy-supportive—in which a parent, partner, or friend doesn't try to be "the boss" but encourages us and helps us make our own choices.[1]

The flip side of the need for autonomy shows itself when our freedom to act and think as we please feels threatened: we experience the urge to protect or restore that freedom. Psychologists call this *reactance*,[2] and it's the source of the "terrible twos" (as well as teenage rebelliousness)—saying "No!" may be the only way toddlers (and sometimes adolescents) know how to assert their own will. But it is also a source of our refusal to accept the imposition of arbitrary limits or unwarranted authority.

Now, most of us do, of course, accept limits on our freedom. We might want to drive 100 miles per hour, or refuse to pay our taxes, or take a week off from work just because we feel like it, yet most of us don't do these things and also don't spend a lot of time thinking or worrying about why we can't. Since we've never believed we were entitled to these freedoms, we generally don't have any trouble accepting those limits without feeling controlled. We're also less likely to take these kinds of restrictions personally; for most of us reactance tends to be triggered not by laws or rules that everyone is expected to follow but by limits or commands directed at us as individuals.

Reactance is especially likely to arise when someone tries to get us to stop doing something that's important to us or tries to pressure us into a change we're not ready for. When we've been exercising our freedom to do what we're accustomed to doing, or just to remain undecided about what to do until we're sure of our decision, our resistance against efforts to force us to change can be intense.

How does reactance affect the way we feel and act? The more reactance we experience, the more *attractive* the threatened way of acting or thinking becomes and the more *hostile* we feel toward the source of the threat.

The effects of external threats to our freedom (often coming from authority figures) tend to be easy to identify. I'm sure you can think of a time when someone told you that you couldn't have something you felt you had a right to—anything from a cigarette to a relationship with someone outside your family's comfort zone. Did you want whatever it was all the

---

[1]Deci, E. L., & Ryan, R. M. (2000). The "what" and "why" of goal pursuits: Human needs and the self-determination of behavior. *Psychological Inquiry, 11*, 227–268.

[2]Brehm, S. S., & Brehm, J. (1981). *Psychological reactance: A theory of freedom and control.* New York: Academic Press.

more? Become more determined to have it? Did you feel resentful or angry toward whoever was restraining you?

The effects of internal threats to our autonomy can be less obvious. For one thing, we usually don't experience reactance when we stop ourselves from doing something that conflicts with a goal that's truly our own. Resisting a cigarette when we're fully committed to quitting smoking or a flirtation when we're committed to monogamy represents "self-control"— it makes us feel *more* autonomous and typically leaves us feeling good about ourselves. But when we're still ambivalent about what we're trying to accomplish, we end up in a battle between the part of ourselves that's doing the controlling and the part that feels controlled. That's when, as you stare at that cigarette you want to smoke or that person you want to ask out, reactance rears its head—the more you tell yourself you're not allowed, the more you want it and the worse you feel.

The Counterproductive Effects of Judgment and Control

Recognizing the need to see ourselves positively teaches us that negative judgment (criticism) shifts our focus away from figuring out what we want or how to get it, to either protecting ourselves against the message that there is something wrong with us or beating ourselves up for not being good enough. Recognizing the need for autonomy teaches us that efforts to control us (demands) intensify our desire to be free from control and divert our energy from dealing with our ambivalence, to fighting off whoever is trying to take away our right and ability to make our own choices.

So the next question to consider is: What does this mean for you?

IS PRESSURE FROM OUTSIDE KEEPING YOU STUCK?

Earlier I told you about an exercise in which professional helpers are asked to think of an area of their own lives where they've been considering a change, and then say for how long they've been considering it. Well, that's not the whole exercise. After they've called out the length of time they've been wrestling with ambivalence, they are asked to consider this scenario, which I'd like you to consider too:

> "Imagine you have to make a decision *right now* about what you're going to do. No more hesitation, no more second thoughts. It's time for a definite, permanent decision, with an unswerving commitment to follow

through and do whatever it takes to make it happen: no excuses, no doubts—full speed ahead."

What is your reaction as you read this? What are you feeling? Thinking? Wanting to say? Write (in your journal or using the online form "Imagine I Had to Decide Right Now" at *www.guilford.com/zuckoff-forms*) whatever comes to mind, without worrying about what it might sound like; just let yourself focus completely on that moment when you're feeling the pressure and then describe it as fully as you can. And please do this before looking ahead at what follows.

Noticing How Pressure from Others Affects You

Most people who do this exercise feel some form of anxiety—from nervousness, tension, or worry to feelings of panic. As discussed in Chapter 1, anxiety is a hallmark of ambivalence, and we spend a lot of time and energy avoiding these unpleasant anxious feelings by trying not to think about the source of our ambivalence. So asking you to think about your ambivalence and then putting pressure on you usually generates and intensifies the anxiety that's lurking in the background.

Anxiety is by no means the only emotion you were likely to feel, though. In fact, when it comes to the kinds of complex and important issues that people get stuck in, they almost always have a variety of reactions to outside pressure to resolve them.

If you focused on the pressure itself, or on its source, you might have felt angry or defiant and rebelled against my authority to force you to decide before you are ready:

- "Where do you get off telling me what to do?"
- "You can say whatever you want; that doesn't mean I'm going to listen."

Or you might have felt attacked and responded by defending or explaining why you can't make that decision right now or why you don't need to change:

- "This isn't a good time for me."
- "I would go ahead, but then it would create all these complications."
- "Things are okay the way they are. I don't really need to deal with this."

Or you might have done a version of the "bobblehead" I wrote about earlier:

- "Yes, okay, sure, I'll go ahead" (all the while knowing that you're not going to do anything at all).

On the other hand, if you focused not on the pressure but on your ambivalence itself, you might have felt helpless or overwhelmed and expected to fail:

- "What am I going to do? This is too much for me to handle."
- "What's the point? Even if I do try, I'm only going to end up back in the same mess."

If so, you might also have begun to beat yourself up for not being able to move ahead:

- "Why can't I just make a decision and stop whining?!"
- "Come on, stupid! Get your act together."

This might quickly have been followed by feelings of *guilt* ("I did something wrong") or *shame* ("There is something wrong with me"):

- "It's my own fault I'm in this situation."
- "I am such a screw-up. What kind of person lets things get so out of control?"

Or you might have felt sad and expressed your grief at the prospect of giving up something that matters to you so you could choose a direction that seems right or desirable:

- "If I do this, it will be so hard on the people I love."
- "How am I going to live without something I've relied on for so long?"

Finally, along with some of these feelings you also might have felt a sense of relief or even excitement at the idea of finally doing *something*. Of course, this feeling also makes sense; if you really could get unstuck and move on with your life, you'd be free of

Motivational speakers inspire people to change . . . until they start thinking for themselves again.

the misery that lingering ambivalence creates. This is why so many people flock to motivational speakers: under the sway of the speaker's persuasive field they believe, in the moment, that they can finally take action, and they often leave inspired. Yet what happens next is almost always just what you'd expect: doubt begins to creep in and discouragement returns as the reality of the decision and what it would mean comes into focus.

This result is similar to what can happen when a person encounters an especially effective salesperson. Many people walk into cosmetics shops, electronics stores, or automobile dealerships with the intention of just looking around but find themselves walking out having bought an expensive package of makeup, a 3-D TV, or even a new car. How does this happen? Usually they've encountered a salesperson who, with a combination of charm, fast talk, and answers for every objection, has persuaded them into a decision they weren't ready to make.

Some of these buyers are relieved. They really wanted that makeup or TV or car but were either afraid to go for it or knew in their hearts that they couldn't quite afford it. The salesperson gave them the push they needed to overcome their hesitation—that is, the push they *wanted* but couldn't quite give themselves. In the whirlwind of the purchase they can rely on the salesperson's enthusiasm to reassure them that they've made the right decision—and if they later have regrets, the salesperson can take the blame and spare them the unpleasant recognition that they made the wrong choice.

On the other hand, many impulse buyers start to have second thoughts from the moment they leave the store: "What was I thinking? How am I going to pay for this? Do I really even want a new car?" Plagued with *buyer's remorse*, they soon look for ways of undoing what they've done.

People who are close to making a major decision but feel afraid to take the risk may well be "convinced" to take the plunge by a firm push. But even among this group, who were not so put off by the pressure (as most ambivalent people are) that they immediately became more resistant, many regret their haste and, feeling unprepared for the new reality they've committed to, renege on the deal, settling back into more or less tortured indecision and resenting the person who almost "made" them decide before they were ready.

So now, please look back at what you wrote in response to the exercise. Which of these reactions did you have?

Defiance and defensiveness, false compliance, expectations of failure, self-abuse, doubt and discouragement, feelings of loss, temporary relief followed by regret (one step forward, two steps back)—what all of these reactions have in common is that they make us *less* ready, willing, and able to choose or to act in a way that leads to sustainable resolution of ambivalence. Rather than move us forward, the demand that we change triggers resistance and leaves us more stuck than before.

Describing the Pressure You're Feeling from Others

Now that you've seen the effects of imaginary pressure to change or make a decision, let's take a look at how pressure from people in your life has actually affected your efforts to address the situation you've been struggling with. As I've said, it's likely that people who want to help have in one way or another been telling you what to do or how to do it. How helpful has that been? What effect has it had? I'd like you to think about the following questions:

- "Who has been a source of pressure to change on the issue I've been struggling with, and what form has that pressure taken? What have these people said or done that's made me feel judged or controlled?"
- "How have the things these people have said or done—no matter how well meaning—affected my efforts to deal with my situation?"

How your companions in ambivalence answered these questions appears below.

. . . .

Pressure from Others about My Dilemma

Alec

Who has pressured me and what have they done?

Most of the pressure is coming from my wife. She gets all moody and cold. When I come home from work after a few drinks with my clients I'll hear, "Why can't you just come home without going to the bar?" And on the weekends it's "Can't you just stay home today?" Trying to make me feel guilty all the time. She refuses to realize that doing my job depends on keeping my connections with my customers strong, and if they want me to meet them on a Saturday for lunch and I say no they might find someone else to buy from.

The other one was my doctor. He made this big deal about how drinking is putting me at risk for a heart attack or stroke or some other big problems, but he was really exaggerating how much I drink.

How has the pressure affected me?

> The more Wendy bugs me, the more I tune her out. I have to admit that the nagging and the guilt make me not want to drink any less because I don't want her to think that I agree with her. As for my doctor, his little speech made me mad, but I don't see him that often, so I can just ignore him.

Barbara

Who has pressured me and what have they done?

> The only person who has any idea that I've been thinking about leaving my husband is my sister, Sue, and she's not the kind of person to tell you what to do. She always sympathizes with how trapped I feel. She also does let me know that she thinks my husband is wonderful—which he is. I don't think it would be fair to describe that as pressure.

How has the pressure affected me?

> When Sue reminds me of how good Steve has been to me, I feel guilty about wanting to leave him. After I talk with her I always come away telling myself that I have to accept that no marriage is perfect. I resolve to let go of my fantasies about starting over, and I feel more settled. But by the next day the feeling of being trapped starts to rise again.

Colin

Who has pressured me and what have they done?

> Paul has a right to complain about my anger, doesn't he? He's a sensitive man. He gets upset when I get angry at him. Afterward, even if I apologize, he will keep bringing it up. But I'm not mad at him for that, or for telling me he can't take it anymore, because I don't think he's trying to control me. He's just worn out. I guess he does judge me, but I can't really blame him for criticizing me for doing something that makes him feel bad, can I?

How has the pressure affected me?

> I honestly don't think I'd be trying to get control of my anger it if it wasn't for Paul. I'm trying to do this for him.

Dana

Who has pressured me and what have they done?

> My family is totally against me studying to become a teacher. They tell me the economy is terrible, and I won't make much money as a teacher even if I do find a job. I wish I could argue with them, but what they're saying is

true. They give me all kinds of good reasons to stay where I am, tell me how mature I've always been, and how they can't understand why suddenly I'm not being sensible.

How has the pressure affected me?

My family is really important to me, and I know they want what's best for me, so I can't just ignore what they say. So I try to tell myself I should be realistic. But I keep thinking about how awesome it would be to be a teacher, and then I have to go into work and deal with all the nonsense there, and that just makes me want it more. I know I shouldn't be thinking that way.

Ellie

Who has pressured me and what have they done?

No one has to put any pressure on me to lose weight. I'm so sick of being fat. The girls at work sometimes tease me about being on another diet, and I laugh it off. Sometimes Gil tries to make me feel better by telling me he loves me no matter what I look like, but that does not help at all.

How has the pressure affected me?

Gil means well, but I get mad at him when he says those things. I feel like he's telling me I should just give up. So I tell myself, I'll show him! It makes me feel like I have to lose weight or I'm a failure. I guess that's pressure I put on myself.

Now it's your turn. Think about anyone who has tried to influence your decision in one direction or another and answer the questions above, using your journal or the online form at *www.guilford.com/zuckoff-forms*. Remember that while some kinds of pressure are obviously negative—for example, being threatened with some kind of punishment if you don't make a change—often the people who care about us pressure us with the best of intentions and in ways that they might not even realize are making us feel pressured.

Reflecting on the Impact of Pressure from Others

Writing about the pressure you feel from others is a good start toward figuring out how to take that pressure off. What strikes you now about what you've just written about pressure from outside, especially in light of what you read earlier about the reasons pressure tends to keep us stuck? Consider your companions' responses before writing your own in your journal or using the form "Reflecting on the Impact of Pressure from Others" at *www. guilford.com/zuckoff-forms*.

- *Alec*: "As long as my wife and my doctor keep making me feel like they're trying to control me, I wouldn't admit that it was a problem even if I thought it was."

- *Barbara*: "It's interesting that whenever I talk to my sister she finds a way to remind me of Steve's good points. It does seem as though she's subtly trying to influence me to stay with him. I don't think she's judging me for how I feel. But maybe she's not really an objective listener?"

- *Colin*: "I didn't think I resented Paul for telling me I need to get control of my anger because I know my anger is hard for him to deal with. But if he wasn't so sensitive, my anger wouldn't be such a problem. Sometimes I do wish he was more like me as far as how I express anger, or even would just accept that for me this is normal."

- *Dana*: "My family wants what's best for me, so I can't be mad at them. But I think that when their voices are running around in my head, it's harder for me to figure out what to do. I wish they would trust me a little more."

- *Ellie*: "Poor Gil, I think he doesn't know what to say to me about my weight. He wants to help, but he really can't win. Maybe I've been letting the girls at work off a little too easy, though. When they make a comment about me dieting it's kind of embarrassing, and that only makes it harder."

IS PRESSURE FROM INSIDE KEEPING YOU STUCK?

Noticing How Pressuring Yourself Affects You

Let's take a closer look at why we may react to external pressure with defiance, anger, or self-justifications but to internal pressure with feelings of failure, guilt and shame, or a sense of hopelessness. When we can't *avoid* the anxiety that surfaces when confronted with an important decision we feel unwilling or unable to make, we look for some way to *reduce* that anxiety, so as not to be made miserable by it. Expressing anger and self-justification toward another person makes us feel powerful instead of vulnerable and distracts us from the fact that we're still stuck. But when there's no one else around to get angry at, we feel trapped. Knowing that if we could only resolve the ambivalence in one direction or the other the anxiety would abate, we turn against ourselves, becoming our own most implacable critic ("What's the matter with you? Stop being so wishy-washy!") and source of pressure to change, decide, or act ("Come on! This cannot be this hard! Can't you just make a decision and do something?").

Of course, then we fight back. The more we try to talk ourselves into doing something we don't want to do, or out of doing something we do want to do, the more we resist being controlled (and dislike ourselves for being the source of the pressure). It's an unwinnable tug-of-war—an irresistible force meeting an immovable object. We also try to defend ourselves against our negative self-judgments, insisting that we're not so bad, telling ourselves we have good reason for not moving forward, or minimizing the importance of doing so. Sometimes that works to get ourselves off our own backs, for a little while. But the main effect of our self-defense is often to trigger an even more vehement attack against ourselves as we redouble our efforts to force ourselves out of the trap we're caught in.

And what a toll that can take! Blaming ourselves for what we now see as the bad choices that got us where we are ("Why am I always putting myself in such a terrible position?"), berating ourselves for being in such a mess ("I hate myself!"), calling ourselves names ("Idiot! Screw-up! Lazy slob! Loser!"), or blistering ourselves with sarcasm ("Great job, genius!")—all of this beating ourselves up is intended to make things better by jolting us out of our complacency or giving ourselves a swift kick in the ass, pushing us from inactivity into action or from waffling into decision. Yet the actual effect is to make us feel even worse about ourselves. Any positive energy we might have for trying to resolve our ambivalence in an effective way—for drawing on our self-knowledge to figure out what we really want for ourselves or our problem-solving abilities to figure out how we can get it—is replaced by thoughts of giving up or feelings of futility. Pretty soon we're feeling guilty for not doing what we should be doing (even if we don't know what that is), helpless to make things better, disgusted about being so stuck and helpless, ashamed of our inadequacy, and maybe also resentful at being made to feel these ways (even if we're doing it to ourselves).

Now, self-persuasion does not *always* generate these kinds of internal reactions. No doubt you can think of times when it's been helpful: standing at the edge of a pool and telling yourself, "I *know* I can make this dive!" or being at a party and saying quietly, as you approach an attractive person, "Just be yourself, relax, smile, what's the worst that can happen?" or sitting at your desk and thinking, "Come on, stay focused, just get through this report, then you can go out and have some fun. . . . ," and so forth.

When we're acting in the service of our own goals, self-talk can be a helpful tool. The things you say to yourself have the quality of positive encouragement, rather than demands to decide or criticism for failing to act. The difference in the effects of this kind of self-persuasion from those that result from self-pressure is stark: increased feelings of being in control and liking yourself versus increasing feelings of being controlled and self-loathing.

You've probably seen depictions of characters stumbling into quick-sand in old movies. The more the hapless victims struggle to escape, the faster they get sucked down. Trying to pressure ourselves into making a decision or changing our situation is a lot like that. A battle that takes place inside our own heads, it produces casualties but no progress, both because of the harm we inflict on ourselves and because when, inevitably, we try to limit the damage by avoiding the whole situation once again, we only find ourselves later up to our necks with no way out and not much energy to try.

Describing Pressure You Put on Yourself in Other Areas of Your Life

Now I'd like to invite you to look at the ways you've been putting pressure on yourself. Because understanding how this affects you is so important, I'd like you first to think about how you've made yourself feel judged or controlled in other areas of your life.

- "When have I put pressure on myself? When I didn't want to make a change or do something but felt like I had to, or had to make a decision but didn't know what the right choice was, or knew what I should do but couldn't get myself to do it, what were the things I said or thought to myself? How did I try to make myself do it? (Did I tell myself I had no choice, threaten myself, imagine what would happen or what others would have thought of me if I didn't?) How do I typically treat myself at those times? (Do I blame, criticize or put myself down, call myself names, or beat myself up?)"

- "What sort of effect has it had when I've pressured myself in these ways? How have I felt about myself? How have I seen myself? What have I felt like doing? What have I actually done?"

How your companions in ambivalence answered these two groups of questions appears on the following page.

Pressure on Myself in Other Areas

Alec

When have I pressured myself and how did I do it?

I'm all about pressure. That's how you make it in my business. Wendy can't seem to get that. You keep pushing even when you don't feel like it, especially when you don't feel like it.

That's what makes this situation at work weird. They're looking for a guy to handle this district that's bigger than mine, and I haven't put myself up for it even though I should. The job has potential for a lot more money. I keep telling myself to go ahead and do it, stop diddling around. So what's my problem? I haven't even asked the regional manager any questions about it. I know I could handle it. I don't know why I'm hesitating.

How has pressuring myself affected my behavior and how I feel about myself?

Normally when I talk to myself that way, it jump-starts me. But none of that has worked this time. It's not like me at all. I've actually told myself a couple of times that I was gonna do it, but then I didn't. I don't even like to admit that. Makes me doubt myself, and that's a real problem. In my line of work, if you're not confident, you're nothing. So yeah, I guess it's making me mad at myself, and no, that's still not getting me to get off my duff and do it.

Barbara

When have I pressured myself and how did I do it?

What comes to mind is the time I was trying to decide whether to finish law school. I'd waited a long time to start. I worked very hard the first two years and I did well. But once I got pregnant again I could tell that Steve was finding it increasingly stressful. He never said anything, but I knew what he wanted me to do. So even though I thought I could find a way to get through the last year, I felt that I had to do what was right for the whole family and not just for me. I told myself that I shouldn't be selfish and that I could always finish later when the timing was better.

How has pressuring myself affected my behavior and how I feel about myself?

My parents taught me that if you're going to do something, do it right. I just accepted that I had to give up something for something else that was more important and that there was nothing to be gained by mooning over it. I loved being a mom, and I wouldn't trade those years when my children were young for anything. I was always taught that you make your decisions and you live with them; you don't indulge yourself in regrets or what-ifs. I never really thought about whether there was a downside to being this way.

Colin

When have I pressured myself and how did I do it?

When I was 15, I got involved with this boy. I loved him, but where we lived it was not safe to be out. Then we broke up, but we stayed connected; we were the only gay kids we knew. Well, he decided to come out, and he wanted me to also. I was definitely not ready, because of the kids at school and my family—I knew they'd go off. He didn't care; he kept saying we had nothing to be ashamed of and if anyone else didn't like it, then the hell with them. I really wasn't ashamed of anything. But he kept calling me a coward, and I started to think maybe he was right—maybe I was just making excuses. So I did it; I came out to my family. And they freaked out exactly the way I knew they would. Everything was different after that, and I was right that it would have been better to wait.

    I know it sounds like I'm talking about what you call "pressure from outside." But really I made me come out, not him. I forced myself to do it even though I didn't want to. And the worst part was, not only did I hurt my family and mess up my high school years, but I hated myself for giving in. I was weak for coming out then, instead of standing up for what I thought was right.

How has pressuring myself affected my behavior and how I feel about myself?

I ended up hating myself. I beat myself up even worse after I came out, for being weak and hurting so many people. But it was confusing because I was also really mad at my parents, because even though I knew they wouldn't be able to handle it I couldn't believe they could treat me that way. So I hated them and I hated myself, and it was like I was in the middle of this maelstrom.

    The whole episode had a big impact on me. For a long time after that I didn't trust anyone because I felt as though everyone who was supposed to care about me had betrayed me. I decided that I was just going to trust myself and not listen to anyone else no matter what. And for a while that's exactly what I did. Which in a way seemed like a good thing, because I knew that I had been right to want to follow my own heart. But that also meant I didn't let anyone in for a long time. And it didn't stop me from beating myself up at other times when I felt like I'd done something stupid or was too afraid to do what I wanted.

Dana

When have I pressured myself and how did I do it?

When I was trying to pick a major in college, my advisor told me to try some different courses. But I felt like I couldn't afford to waste any time. I was there to get a degree that would get me a good job. So even though I liked English and psychology better, I declared a major in business as soon I could. But instead of doing my accounting homework I'd be writing a poem. When I started working at a childcare center I'd spend hours thinking about what kind of craft I could do with the kids. I would lecture myself a lot, like, "You're not spending all this money so you can make minimum wage. You have to focus on what's important." I'd remind myself of what I could have once I went to work for real. I didn't usually beat myself up, but I did call myself "flaky" to my friends.

How has pressuring myself affected my behavior and how I feel about myself?

Well, the stuff I did worked; I did get a good job right out of college when a lot of people ended up back home with their parents. But I'd also be very frustrated with myself because I daydreamed and took too long to get things done. Sometimes I'd feel like a fraud because I had to work so hard to focus, as if I were working against something blocking me. (That's also partly why I didn't really think about grad school.) And sometimes I still feel that way because my friends and my family all think I have it so together and I'm so mature when I feel like I'm not really going anywhere in my career and I'm less and less happy with it.

Ellie

When have I pressured myself and how did I do it?

When we were first married, I thought it would be nice to bring Gil's family and my family all together for Thanksgiving. Somehow this turned into me hosting both families every year. But now the family is twice as large, and I'm older and working and taking care of my kids. By the time I was pregnant with my 9-year-old I'd had it. But I would tell myself that traditions are so important to the family, my sister is not much of a cook, and my mom's getting older, so how could I not do it? And it is a nice occasion every year, even if I don't get to spend much time with everyone because I'm so busy in the kitchen. So when I feel resentful, I just tell myself this is what holds a family together, don't be selfish. I also do think of asking for some help, but then I think it's no big deal and no one else does things exactly the way I do them, so I'll get by for another year.

How has pressuring myself affected my behavior and how I feel about myself?

The truth is I don't get much joy from having the family at Thanksgiving anymore. I used to be very proud of myself, but now after spending every night after work for a week baking and cleaning, I barely get everything on the table. Honestly I can't even care that much how much everyone's enjoying it, but that makes me feel like a terrible person. A few times I let slip some little comments about how much I'm doing, but then I felt even more

> *guilty. Now I start to dread the holiday coming when fall rolls around, and I never felt that way years ago.*

Now it's your turn. Think about how you make yourself feel judged or controlled in your life in general and answer the questions above, in your journal or using the form at *www.guilford.com/zuckoff-forms*.

Reflecting on the Impact of Pressure You Put on Yourself in Other Areas of Your Life

What stands out to you now about what you've just written about pressure from inside, especially in light of what you read earlier? Consider your companions' responses before writing your own in your journal or using the form "Reflecting on Pressure I Put on Myself in Other Areas of My Life" at *www.guilford.com/zuckoff-forms*:

- *Alec:* "I didn't agree with what you were saying about how putting pressure on yourself gets in the way. I'm still not sure it's making me more stuck. But I have to admit that it's not working this time, and it bothers me that I can't figure out why."

- *Barbara:* "It's hard to admit how disappointed I was to give up becoming a lawyer, because it still feels selfish to think that way. I can't imagine not having been there through my kids' childhoods, but I don't think I want to go on making choices that way, by being 'practical,' which always means making the sacrifice."

- *Colin:* "Pushing yourself do something can seem like a good idea because it makes you stop going around in your head, but then you can regret your decision and realize you weren't thinking clearly, even though you thought you were. I was surprised at how strong the feelings are now. I think I'm still hurting from what happened."

- *Dana:* "I always thought my problem was not being able to make myself overcome my flakiness. It's still hard for me to see how lecturing myself could have made it worse. But I have to admit that it hasn't made me feel very good about myself."

- *Ellie:* "I miss the way I used to feel about the holidays, and I don't like to think about how much that's changed. Even if it's because I keep making myself do it even though I don't want to, I don't know how I could stop without feeling awful. Then again, it seems pretty goofy to say I want help and then tell myself I don't need it."

Describing the Pressure You Put on Yourself about Your Dilemma

Now that you've given some thought to the ways you put pressure on yourself from inside, let's focus on how this affects your struggle with your dilemma. Please ask yourself the following questions about how you've made yourself feel judged or controlled:

- "How have I been putting pressure on myself to change, make a decision, or take action on the issue I'm stuck in? What are the things I say to myself when I start thinking about the issue? (Do I tell myself I have no choice, threaten myself, imagine what will happen or what others will think of me?) How do I treat myself at those times? (Do I blame, criticize or put myself down, call myself names, or beat myself up?)"

- "What sort of effect has pressuring myself in these ways had on me? When I think about the issue I'm stuck in, how do I feel about myself? How do I see myself? What do I feel like doing? What do I actually do?"

How your companions answered the questions appears below.

. . . .
Pressure on Myself about My Dilemma

Alec

What have I done to pressure myself?

> My only dilemma has been how to get my wife off my case. I haven't been thinking seriously about cutting down. It would be nice if she'd let me do my own thinking about it for a change.

How has pressuring myself affected my behavior and how I feel about myself?

> Mostly I want my wife to leave me alone. I admit that my buddy's heart problem gave me a jolt, but that didn't make me feel bad about myself; it just made me think a little.

Barbara

What have I done to pressure myself?

> Most of the time I try to put it out of my mind or tell myself to stop being a fool. No one gets to have it all. Many people would be thrilled to have my

life. So I tell myself to stop being greedy. I remind myself what a good man Steve is and how lucky I am to have him.

I think I've known all along that my sister isn't really a neutral listener. I've been using her to help keep myself in line. Because these feelings I'm having are terrifying. Who do I think I am? I'm not as sharp as I used to be, and I'm not nearly as attractive. Why can't I get control of myself? The urge to leave is so powerful sometimes I feel like I'll die if I don't act on it. There must be something wrong with me. Am I a bad person after all? Am I sick—do I need medication? Is it just menopause and hormones? I picture the pain on Steve's face, how horribly betrayed my children would feel, and I hate myself for even thinking about doing such a terrible thing to them. But none of that stops me from wanting something more so badly I can almost taste it.

How has pressuring myself affected my behavior and how I feel about myself?

I am so angry at myself for not being able to stop obsessing about this. I am a grown woman, but I feel like a crazy person. I'm so disappointed in myself, more than anything. I thought I knew who I was. My life made sense. Now I feel like I want to run away from it all, the thoughts going around and around in my head like the gerbils the kids had, running on their wheels and getting nowhere. That's when I call my sister and let her make me feel guilty. Then I feel stronger for a little while, more like myself, and I tell myself that I really am going to start acting my age. Which usually lasts until the next day, when the whole thing starts all over again.

Colin

What have I done to pressure myself?

I always felt bad after I got really mad at Paul. But I guess I also felt he wasn't seeing my side, and that would make anyone mad. So for a long time I didn't really try to control my anger with him. But since he told me he can't stay with me unless I do, I've been talking to myself a lot. I tell myself that it shouldn't be so hard. I think about how much I love him and that I don't want to lose him. I remind myself of how lonely I was before we got together and how much I hated dating and hook-ups. I think of how stupid it is to jeopardize what we have. I go over all these thoughts in my head again and again to try to make sure that I don't get sloppy and forget.

Most of all I tell myself not to get mad about things and promise myself I will not yell and that I will not lose control. I think about different techniques like walking away instead of getting loud, or counting backward from 10 to 0, or taking deep breaths, and I promise myself that I will use them when I get mad.

How has pressuring myself affected my behavior and how I feel about myself?

> So far it hasn't been working. To be honest, I've been telling myself for a while that it's time to get serious, but I'm still not keeping myself under control very well. Just lately I've started to feel a little lame, like why am I still blowing up? Thinking about that makes me want to try harder. And I do, but I still lash out—sometimes over nothing.
>
> I also have to admit I have been feeling irritated with Paul for making such a big deal out of this. It feels a little unfair that I'm the one who has to do all the changing. I guess I'm a little confused about who's right and who's wrong. Then again, I can start to feel pretty bad about myself. A couple of times I've gone off by myself and cried because I felt kind of hopeless.

Dana

What have I done to pressure myself?

> I tell myself all the reasons I shouldn't go against my parents' wishes and throw away what I've worked so hard for. There's no way to know for sure I'd be happy teaching. Maybe I idealized being a teacher, and when you actually teach every day it gets boring and frustrating just like my job is now. Maybe I'm just someone who will never be satisfied, no matter what I do.
>
> So then I get mad at myself for wasting time looking online at grad schools. I didn't realize it, but I do a lot of the same things I did when I was in college, telling myself to stop being flaky and irresponsible and reminding myself about the good things about my job. But now I've got even more ammunition, because my family is used to having my financial support, and I can tell myself that it would be selfish to jerk the rug out from under their feet.

How has pressuring myself affected my behavior and how I feel about myself?

> It's interesting—this time it's not working like it did in college. Even though I'm even harder on myself now than I was then, I'm still surfing the Web for teaching programs and imagining what it would be like to have my own classroom. I'm mostly confused and stressed and overwhelmed. I've been feeling nervous, and sometimes I get these panicky feelings, and my heart starts to pound, and I feel lightheaded. One thing's for sure, trying not to think about it seems to be pretty futile.

Ellie

What have I done to pressure myself?

> Every morning I tell myself I'm going to stick to my diet. All I have to do is look at my fat clothes to feel disgusted with myself. I have motivation all

around me—TV, magazines, and all these other women who have nice figures and self-control. And I'm pretty good all day. But by lunchtime I'm thinking about dinner for my family. Then I'm stressed about being in the kitchen for hours so everyone can have what they want. I'm hungry and tired, and I'm nibbling and tasting my way through the night. I get disgusted and I start telling myself what a poor excuse for an adult I am. Oh yeah, I can really use some choice words about myself when I'm stuffing myself. I hate how little control I have! Then I tell myself that I'll start fresh tomorrow, I guess to stop myself from feeling so horrible and try to have some hope.

How has pressuring myself affected my behavior and how I feel about myself?

I've been at this for longer than I want to think about, and I keep gaining weight. I feel like a total failure. I can hardly stand to get on the scale because when I see the number I want to scream. I feel like I've let down Gil—he has to live with a fat wife. It's enough to make me feel so desperate that I start thinking about extreme measures, like I should get my jaw wired shut or get my stomach stapled or who knows what. Then I swing the other way and think it's completely hopeless. I should just give up and try to accept that I'll be overweight for the rest of my life, and Gil should accept that, too. I can even start to resent him, which is crazy, because he's not the one telling me that I'm a worthless wife.

Now it's your turn. Think about how putting pressure on yourself has affected you and your struggle with your dilemma and answer the questions above, either in your journal or using the form at *www.guilford.com/zuckoff-forms.*

Reflecting on the Impact of the Pressure You Put on Yourself about Your Dilemma

What stands out to you now about what you've just written about pressure from inside, especially in light of what you read earlier about the reasons pressure tends to keep us stuck? Consider your companions' responses before writing your own in your journal or using the form "Reflecting on Pressure I Put on Myself about My Dilemma" at *www.guilford.com/zuckoff-forms:*

- *Alec:* "Like I said, the pressure that's been affecting me when it comes to drinking has been from my wife, mostly. But obviously her hassling me hasn't given me much space to think about it for myself or decide what I want to do, if anything."

- *Barbara*: "I'm actually a bit shocked at how harshly I've been thinking about myself. It's as if I'm so disoriented by the feelings I'm having that I can't get my footing. It does seem clear that being angry and impatient with myself and ordering myself to set all my feelings aside has not gotten me any closer to getting this resolved."

- *Colin*: "I think I'm more upset about this than I've wanted to admit. It's not comfortable to be the one who has the problem. I'm not completely sure that Paul's 100% right and I'm 100% wrong. But I really don't understand why I don't seem to be able to do better at it once I set my mind to it. I guess that's also a little bit scary."

- *Dana*: "I went through this big battle with myself in college, and I thought I was done with it, but now here it is again. Only this time I don't just have to discipline myself until I graduate—there's no end in sight unless I can talk some sense into myself once and for all. But this time I don't seem to have much sense."

- *Ellie*: "I'm not sure what's worse—how overweight I am or failing at diet after diet and being so angry at myself. I'm like a rat in a maze. It has to stop."

YOU DON'T HAVE TO CHANGE

Exploring the pressure you've been under has most likely made at least one thing obvious: If pressure from outside or inside were going work, it would have already. But no one wants to be judged, and no one wants to feel controlled. No matter what sort of pressure might be brought to bear, we insist on our *right* to remain undecided or to maintain the status quo until we know what we want; we insist on our *inability* to choose or to make the change we've been thinking (and stressing) about until and unless we truly come to believe that it's possible for us. When someone (including ourselves) judges or tries to control us, we feel psychologically threatened; when we feel threatened, our focus turns to protecting ourselves—in this case, our good feelings about ourselves, and our freedom to make our own choices. And when we're busy protecting ourselves, we aren't making changes or decisions.

So telling you "You don't have to change" does not just recognize a fact; it expresses a guiding philosophy and a commitment. You don't *have to* deal with the issue, make a decision, or take any action right now, no matter who has been telling you that you do. No one can make you—not the people in your life, not me, and not even you. You could choose to do nothing or keep going the way you are, either because you don't yet know what you want or don't know if you can get it or both, or because you decide that keeping things the same is actually the right choice for you. That is your right. And more than that, all the attempts (your own as well as others') to *force* you do something before you're ready are actually making it *harder* for you to come to a decision or feel able to accomplish what you want to accomplish.

Whether or not you make any change is completely up to you. This is *your* life, and you are the one who will live with whatever decision you make or solution you come to, whenever you come to it. It's only right that you should be the one who decides and that you should do so when you're ready and not before. The choice and the timing are yours; no one and nothing can change that, *and that's as it should be.* So before we talk any more about the possibility of change, let's take the pressure off.

3

The Other Side
of the Pressure Paradox

Sheila was a woman in her 40s whose husband, Tom, was pleasant and reliable—except when, every few months, he would go on a bender. For years Sheila joined him in these drinking binges. Through her work in therapy with me she had decided to stop, but she felt some trepidation about how Tom might react. Her fears were confirmed soon enough—one memorable day Sheila came to my office wearing a pair of dark glasses, beneath which she revealed an ugly black eye.

My response was immediate. I went into "crisis" mode, emphasizing the need to ensure that Sheila was safe from any more violence—a conviction that was only strengthened when she revealed that Tom was still drinking and this was not the first time he had hit her while under the influence. I offered options to get her out of the house at least temporarily and named a women's shelter I could refer her to. I warned that Tom would no doubt express remorse when he sobered up, but that clinical experience indicated that this would make it no less likely that he would hit her again in the future. I did everything I could to persuade Sheila of the need to separate herself from her abuser.

But Sheila's responses to my exhortations were strikingly consistent: to every point I made she replied with a reason why she need not or could not leave. Most of the time Tom was a loving husband and a good father, and these incidents were so infrequent, she said. She had stopped working to stay home and raise their child and had no idea how she would support herself and her son on her own. Moving to another part of town would mean a new school for her son and disruption of his life. Everything she owned was in the house, and there would be no way to leave without Tom knowing about it, which he might react to by attacking her again. And despite what he had done, she insisted, she still loved him, and she was not ready to give up on the marriage.

I began to grow impatient; I was trying to help keep Sheila safe, yet she seemed determined to thwart my efforts. I became increasingly aware that we were getting nowhere. I began to question Sheila's judgment and to consider dropping the subject.

And then I realized that Sheila was not the problem in the conversation; I was. I thought about what Sheila had been saying. I considered what it might be like to face the prospect of turning a life you'd built for two decades upside down. And I said, "Sheila, as I think about the things you've been telling me, all of the reasons for not leaving the situation you're in, it seems the decision that's making the most sense for you right now is just to stay where you are."

Sheila listened intently as I spoke. When I finished, she paused, fixed me with an unblinking stare, and replied, with vehemence, "Are you nuts?"

And then she went on to tell me all the reasons for leaving. When it came to getting hit by her husband, even once was too much. She'd supported herself before, and she could do it again if she had to. It was worse for her son to be exposed to his father's violence toward her than it would be for him to have to change schools. She might lose some of her stuff, but that was a small price to pay compared with the risk of getting hurt. Going to a shelter, if it came to that, would be hard to take, but it wouldn't be permanent, and she'd made it through worse. Most of all, what kind of love is it if you have to live in fear?

Sheila went on this way, speaking firmly and with conviction, for several minutes as I sat and listened. Every argument I could have thought of to persuade her to leave came tumbling out of her without another word from me.

Ultimately, Sheila decided she did not want to continue the marriage. She did not decide to leave Tom that day; despite her awareness of the many reasons to leave and her belief that she could find a way to manage it, she felt she needed more time to think about what taking such a drastic step would mean for her life as a whole. But by the end of that session she found herself (she said) thinking more clearly, and she formulated a plan to keep herself safe at home until her husband sobered up and then talk to him about what had happened.

So what does this have to do with you? What happened between Sheila and me reveals the other side of the pressure paradox: While pressure to change keeps people stuck, *acceptance* frees people for change.

Initially it had seemed to me that Sheila was determined to stay with her husband. Yet my judgment was wrong. Sheila was *ambivalent* about her situation. She was already aware of good reasons for leaving Tom. But when she contemplated acting on those reasons, she became equally aware of important concerns that taking that step seemed to ignore.

So Sheila came to see me that day in the middle of an extended argument *with herself* about the situation she was facing. After all, she was a bright and self-respecting woman whose husband had hit her in a drunken rage. How could she *not* have been wrestling with what to do, weighing her options, and struggling to decide what the right choice was for her?

Unfortunately, Sheila's argument with herself was not getting her anywhere; oscillating in her own mind between why she should leave and why she should stay, she was trapped in a frustrating cycle of internal conflict, anxiety, and self-blame. Picture an old-fashioned scale, with reasons to leave on one side and reasons to stay on the other. From Sheila's perspective, the two sides of the scale were balanced and she could not move in either direction.

By now you probably recognize my mistake. Sheila was not about to let me tip the scale with arguments she'd already been making (and disputing) to herself. However unintentionally, my responses implied that her reasons for staying were not worth taking seriously and that her fears about leaving were inconsequential. As long as Sheila experienced me as trying to persuade her to leave her husband, she felt compelled to argue against it.

Only when I stopped trying to persuade Sheila to do what *I* thought she should do and began instead to understand and accept her concerns, did the conversation become constructive. Sheila no longer had to defend herself against the hurtful message that there was something wrong with her for having stayed through years of binges and occasional violence—a message that echoed and amplified thoughts she was already having about herself. She no longer had to defend her freedom to make her own decision against my efforts to direct her actions. Suddenly she could tell me her reasons for leaving and her fears about staying—thoughts and feelings that she'd never spoken aloud *for fear that whoever was listening would try to use her own words to push her into a change she wasn't ready for.* And once she had put all those thoughts into words, she found herself thinking differently about her situation, with a freshness and clarity that allowed her to see a way forward.

> People won't say what they think when they expect their words to be used against them.

ACCEPTANCE FACILITATES CHANGE

Acceptance is the experience of feeling deeply understood, valued, and affirmed in who we are, rather than needing to be different to feel worthwhile. It's a sense of trust in ourselves and confidence that our choices will be treated with respect. When we feel accepted and accept ourselves as we are, we no longer have to focus our mental and emotional energy on protecting ourselves against negative judgment, control, and the bad feelings they cause in us. Instead, our energy and focus are freed to address the questions "Where do I go from here? How can I grow further?"[1] And that's when change, or just coming to a decision about what's right for us, becomes an inviting possibility rather than a heavy burden or painful obligation.

Acceptance, in turn, requires compassion—openness to the suffering of others and the desire to alleviate it with kindness and care. Compassion includes the awareness that we are all courageous in facing challenges and making decisions without knowing with certainty whether things will turn out right, but also fallible and flawed, bound to make mistakes and even do harm despite our good intentions. The acceptance and understanding created by this awareness promote the willingness to forgive those failings in others, and also, crucially, in ourselves. As psychologist Kristin Neff[2] has emphasized, *self-compassion*—concern for our own suffering and struggles, kindness to ourselves as a way of alleviating them, and nonjudgmental acceptance of our limits as human beings—is a core component of well-being and positive growth.

Increasing our experience of acceptance and compassion from others and from ourselves frees us to think with a clear mind and to devote our energy to solving the problem at hand instead of defending ourselves against the sources of pressure. It restores our sense of autonomy, and when we feel in control of our own decisions and actions, rather than feeling controlled by others or by our own demanding inner voice, we are better able to see ourselves and our situation clearly and tap into our natural ability to identify what is best for us according to our own lights. Reducing our impatience and frustration with ourselves and allowing us to forgive rather than castigate ourselves for our hesitancy and wrong turns opens up a space

---

[1]Rogers, C. R. (1961). On becoming a person: A therapist's view of psychotherapy. Boston: Houghton Mifflin.

[2]Neff, K. (2003). Self-compassion: An alternative conceptualization of a healthy attitude toward oneself. *Self and Identity, 2,* 85–101.

for honest and calm reflection that can produce our best thinking about how to resolve our dilemmas.

This, then, is my goal for the rest of this chapter: to guide you through to the other side of the pressure paradox by helping you achieve the acceptance and compassion that will allow you to begin moving forward.

GAINING ACCEPTANCE AND COMPASSION

Acceptance and Compassion from People Who Have Pressured You

In the section "Describing the Pressure You're Feeling from Others" in Chapter 2, you wrote about people in your life who have been telling you what you should do and giving you the message that your reasons for wanting or not wanting to change were misguided or not worth taking seriously. Chances are these people believe they're doing their best to help you. If they suddenly started "telling you what you want to hear instead of what you *need* to hear," they might worry that they'd just be "enabling" you to go on acting in ways they're sure aren't good for you. So we can't really expect them to change their approach.

But what if they *could* understand that what they've been doing has been working against you and knew what really *would* be the best thing they could do? If they care about you, they probably would want you to hear whatever they could say to help take the pressure off. And because you know better than anyone else exactly what that would sound like, you're the perfect person to say to yourself what they don't know how to say to you.

What would it sound like if, instead of putting pressure on you, the people in your life said exactly what you'd want them to say? What your companions imagined hearing appears below.

. . . .

What I'd Most Want to Hear from People Who Have Pressured Me

Alec

I'd want her to show some sign of appreciating everything I've done for our family. It's like she doesn't realize the pressure I'm under. . . . I'd want her to say that she gets that I work damn hard, and it isn't easy for me to schmooze customers and be funny when I know what's at stake. Just once I'd like to hear her say, "Do what you need to do, honey. I know that everything you do is for me and Jen. If having a few drinks is part of what it takes, then

I understand." I know she worries about my health, I know she wishes I was around more, but if she could just see how she makes things harder on me! Like at the end of a day, if she would just say, "I'm sorry for nagging you. If you really needed to come home late to do your job, then okay." I don't expect her to be completely fine with it; I just need her to back off. And I'd love to hear after a long night, "I'm glad you're home."

Barbara

Well, I did have the thought once, more like a momentary fantasy when I was feeling desperate, that somehow it would make a big difference if my sister would say something like, "Sis, it's true that I love Steve. But I grew to love him because he loves you and has tried to make you happy. If you're not, then what I want the most is for you to find your spark again. I'd be lying if I said I wouldn't miss you two as a couple, but this isn't about me. I'd much rather see you more yourself again, and if you can't get back there married to Steve, then whatever it takes is what I want you to do. I'll be right beside you all the way."

Colin

I have to admit I'd love to hear him say I don't need to make any major changes because he's realized my anger isn't that bad. Something like "It isn't such a big deal. We've both lost our temper, and there were times when you had every right to be mad about the way you'd been treated. We do anger differently, but that doesn't mean there's anything wrong with the way you do it. You're entitled to be the way you are, even if I don't always like it. I can be too sensitive sometimes. We each have our share of the blame in how things have gone wrong. Let's just go back to the way we were and both try to make things better between us."

Dana

I guess it would feel a lot better if they could say to me that it is my choice, and if I want to try to do something like working with children they think I'd be pretty good at it. That I deserve to follow my dreams. It would be good if they could see that playing it safe isn't all there is to life. I can accept that they think it makes sense for me to stay where I am. I just wish they could also see that there are other things besides money that I don't have. I'd love for them to be able to say, "You are young. If you don't take risks now, you never will. . . . Sometimes in life people have to take a step backward to move forward." And "Don't worry. You've been helping carry us for long enough. We'll be okay if this is what you decide to do." And "It's up to you. We know you'll make the right decision. We trust you."

Ellie

Usually I think there's nothing anyone can say that I haven't already heard, and if they did come up with something new it wouldn't help anyway. I guess Gil could say he'd be willing to help out to make my life easier day to day. He doesn't understand how hard it is to control my eating when I'm so tired and stressed. I wish he understood how bad it feels that I can't seem to succeed no matter what. I know he loves me, and he never complains, but it might feel good if he said, "Honey, I can see how hard this is for you and how much it matters to you. If there's any way that I can help you out, I want to, and I'll get the kids to help too." Even though I would feel too guilty to take him up on the offer it might be nice to hear.

As for my friends, if just one of them could say to me, "You deserve a pat on the back!" As a matter of fact, if anyone at all came up to me and said, "You work so hard taking care of other people, you're a great wife and mother—by the time you're done at the end of the day it's no wonder you're too exhausted to think about watching what you eat. You deserve to eat something good!" I know that isn't a good excuse and that kind of thinking won't get me anywhere, but a lot of times I feel like I'm swimming upstream, and when it seems like people think I'm just floating along I feel pretty bad about myself.

Now it's your turn. Imagine what the people who have been putting pressure on you would say if they understood how important it was to take the pressure off and knew how to help you feel understood and accepted. Remember, this is not what they would say to you in reality; if you notice that you're imagining them giving you advice or that you feel criticized, blamed, or bad about yourself as you're writing, stop and think about a time when you felt really understood and accepted by someone. Then imagine what someone could say that would make you feel that way right now. Enter your thoughts in your journal or use the form at *www.guilford.com/ zuckoff-forms*.

Giving Acceptance to Someone in Your Shoes

Coming to feel accepted instead of pressured by others is half the battle of taking the pressure off. Accepting and expressing compassion for yourself, rather than criticizing yourself for being stuck or demanding of yourself that you change or decide before you know what you want or how to get there, is the other half and, as we saw in Chapter 2, the more difficult to accomplish. Once we've convinced ourselves of our own inadequacy, it's hard to see ourselves differently.

So let's try something a little bit easier. Imagine that someone you care about is stuck in the same dilemma that you're currently struggling with. Imagine that you want to help that person feel deeply understood and valued just as he (or she) is in the situation, rather than judged for what he is lacking or hasn't done; trusted to make his own decisions in his own time, rather than needing to act now or allow someone else to tell him what to do. How could you help your friend feel that way?

What your companions imagined themselves saying appears below.

. . . .

What I'd Say to Help Someone
in My Shoes Feel Accepted and Understood

Alec

First I'd say, "You bust your butt for your family because you love them. You're not out until all hours having fun; you're doing what you need to do to take care of them. I know it's a sacrifice missing out on your kid growing up and there are plenty of times you'd rather be home. But your wife needs to realize she wouldn't have half of what she has if you didn't do what you do." Then I'd say, "I think your wife loves you and you know that deep down. The problem is she doesn't show it and that makes you feel like she doesn't appreciate you. Maybe she nags you so much because she worries about you. She probably doesn't mean to add extra stress to your life. But the bottom line is that she makes you feel like you're wrong. And alcohol or no alcohol, you're a hard worker and good husband, and you deserve to feel like she gets that and trusts you to make the right decisions for you and for your family."

Barbara

I'd say to my friend that this is a very difficult situation you are in and I want you to know that I understand. It may look from the outside that you'd be a fool to give up what you have and that it would be selfish to hurt the people you love for no good reason and you'd only regret it. But they don't know what this is like for you on the inside. You're not trying to feel this way—you've been trying very hard not to. And I know what it's like to feel so alone with these strange, stubborn feelings that just won't go away. I don't know what the answer is, but I guess I can tell you that you're not bad or crazy because I'm going through this, too. So maybe we need to stop fighting this thing and pay attention to what it might mean for us. You don't deserve to feel so terrible, and whatever you decide to do, your heart is in the right place.

Colin

"You are not the kind of man who would threaten the person you love, and I know you'd never hit anyone in anger. It's not fair for you to take all the blame. So I'm sure you feel backed into a corner and it's hard to understand why he's doing this. And you must feel really bad to be seen in such a negative way by the person you've chosen to spend your life with. But I also know that what you've wanted all along is for the two of you to be happy. So maybe this is what it takes. Maybe the way you get angry has affected him more than you ever realized. Maybe loving him means looking at this from a fresh angle. I'm not telling you to just grit your teeth and change. I'm starting to realize that's not going to work. But I guess it really is up to you to decide whether this is worth it to you, to see him happy and for him to want to stay."

Dana

I would say to her, "You love your family very much, and you want to be a good daughter. It is great that you have worked so hard to become independent. You had to make some sacrifices to get where you are, so you should feel proud of yourself. You have proven that you are responsible and mature. But those things are not from doing this one job; they are qualities that you possess. People don't know what it feels like to feel underestimated and to know there's no real challenge left for you. Your parents might actually get the first point since they raised you not to allow others to talk down to you. From their viewpoint, it is a lot to give up for such a risky road, and in many ways they are right. But you have had this wish for so long and you can imagine yourself feeling fulfilled and happy doing it. So neither choice would mean that you are irresponsible or immature."

Ellie

I think I'd say, "It's hard for people who don't have a weight problem to understand how frustrating and difficult it is. It would be nice if people were less judgmental. People seem to think it's not so hard—just get some self-control and don't be so weak. And then other people think we should just live with it, or, even worse, sometimes they pity us. I really feel for you having to act like none of that stuff bothers you when it really hurts.

Sometimes we end up being our own worst enemies, though, don't we? I know you get mad and say mean things to yourself, and that really doesn't help. You could probably say more nice things to yourself, like you are not a total failure just because you're heavy. I'm not telling you what to say to yourself, I'm just saying you deserve to hear that. You have a very loving family and good friends and a pretty good sense of humor. You wouldn't have all that if you were so worthless. Your weight isn't everything. We both *need to stop judging ourselves and stop letting other people's opinions affect us so much. I don't think either of us is gonna be able to figure anything else out until we stop that."*

• •

Now it's your turn. What would *you* say to help a friend who was struggling with the same situation as you feel completely accepted? Write your answers in your journal or use the form at *www.guilford.com/zuckoff-forms*. Don't be surprised if, like Colin and Ellie, you feel tempted to give a little advice or tell your friend what to do. After all, that's what you've been hearing from others and, very likely, from yourself. If you find yourself giving advice, pause for a moment and remind yourself that your aim is to convey acceptance and compassion and nothing more. If you're not sure how your words would be taken, ask yourself, "How would I feel if someone said that to me?" If the answer is "Blamed" or "Judged" or just "Not too good," try to write something instead that *would* make you feel understood in a good way.

Remember, the goal of this activity is not for you to resolve your own ambivalence. Don't use this activity to put more pressure on yourself; use it to set those expectations aside and express the kindness you feel toward a person you care about.

Reflecting on Acceptance and Compassion Received and Given

After some thinking and writing, a little time for reflection can bring a fresh perspective. Please reread the response you wrote to the first of these two activities. Then I'd like you to do something different with the second.

You might remember that I said in the Prelude that there would be times when I would ask you to read aloud something you've written. It turns out that the part of our brains that processes sounds—including speech—is closely linked to the part that is responsible for storing memories of events we have experienced. This is not an accident; from the time humans developed the capacity for language we have told each other the stories of our lives, not only as a way of sharing them with others but also as a way of knowing ourselves. We also have new evidence[3] that hearing our own voices activates our brains in specific ways that help to resolve ambivalence. So please read your response to the second activity out loud

---

[3]Feldstein Ewing, S. W., Yezhuvath, U., Houck, J. M., & Filbey, F. M. (2014). Brain-based origins of change language: A beginning. *Addictive Behaviors, 39,* 1904–1910.

and listen to yourself as you do so. Here's what struck your companions when they read theirs:

- *Alec:* "I didn't realize how much it bothers me that my wife doesn't show me any appreciation these days. When we got married, she told me all the time what a great provider I was, and I was making a lot less money. Now she's always talking about feeling lonely and missing how I used to be and I don't like any of that."

- *Barbara:* "I'm realizing how hard it's been to feel alone with all of these thoughts and feelings churning inside me. Imagining my sister saying those things makes me aware of missing her being that way. Now she's like my guilty conscience instead of my emotional support. Also, when I realize that I haven't been trying to feel this way, I've been trying to stop feeling this way, I don't feel so guilty and ungrateful as I usually do about being dissatisfied even though I have so much."

- *Colin:* "It sounds like I think the whole problem is his fault and I'm the victim. I know that's not true. I start to feel like all the blame is being put on me, and then I want to put all the blame on him. But it doesn't help to blame each other, because then everyone feels bad, and the point is for both of us to feel better. Somehow you have to find a way to admit your part of the problem and try to change it. But you have to do that without feeling like a horrible person."

- *Dana:* "One moment I'm telling myself that I need to stop this nonsense, and the next moment I'm talking about my parents telling me to take risks and follow my dreams. It's hard for me not to get mad at myself for being so indecisive. But it felt good to hear myself saying to 'a friend' that 'she' has a lot to be proud of and it's not so strange that 'she's' confused. No one tells me it's a tough decision; they just tell me that I'm crazy for considering it. And of course I tell myself the same thing."

- *Ellie:* "I liked imagining my husband saying he wants to help. But then I felt scared, and I don't know why. Same with the girls at work; I liked imagining them saying those nice things to me, but then for some reason I felt bad about it afterward. When it was a 'friend' I was talking to, I could understand how hard it was for her and I really wanted to help her feel better. But when my mind switched over to it being me, I didn't feel that way anymore. I guess I'm pretty good at helping a friend. I'm not so good at believing it myself, though."

Now it's your turn. What stood out for you when you reread aloud what you had written? What did you find interesting or surprising? What did it make you think or feel? (Write your answers in your journal or use the form "Reflecting on Acceptance and Compassion Received and Given" at *www.guilford.com/zuckoff-forms*.)

One more step now. Please reread the reflection you just wrote and see what you notice about the way you thought and felt about yourself when writing it. Here's what your companions found:

- *Alec:* "I guess I sound pretty ticked off at my wife. Maybe I don't like admitting how much it matters to me that she doesn't tell me good things about myself anymore. But I also feel like she's questioning my judgment. And maybe that bothers me, especially because I've been having some doubts about myself, which I also don't like to admit. Like that situation with the promotion, it's got me rattled, and that's not good."

- *Barbara:* "I think I make myself feel guilty to keep myself in line and stop me from acting selfishly. But I'm also noticing that wanting something I'm missing makes me think of myself as selfish. I've always thought that was true, but now I'm not sure."

- *Colin:* "I was critical of myself for sounding like I thought I was innocent. But I was also kind to myself by saying that it's not a good idea to make myself choose which of us is the bad one. It's really hard for me not to focus on figuring out who's to blame, though. Probably the truth is it's both. Or maybe the idea is to stop looking to blame anybody. I just know that if I'm the one who has to do all the changing, that means I'm the one who's been all wrong. I can't believe that, so I've been trying to change when part of me feels like it's unfair for the whole burden to be on me. Which might help to explain why I've been so bad at it so far. (Oops, another criticism.)"

- *Dana:* "I see frustration at myself for not being able to stop going in circles. But mainly I've been trying to convince myself that I just have to figure out how to stop my foolishness. Yet that's not true. I might be crazy for considering going back to school, but I can't keep pretending that I don't have a decision to make, because I do. It's just that I can't even tell whether I'd want to take the risk because I keep telling myself it's not even supposed to be a choice. I'm not going to be able to think clearly about this whole situation until I stop telling myself that."

- *Ellie:* "I can see pretty clearly that I'm not very kind or understanding toward myself. Or it's more than that—when someone says something nice to me, I push it away, and that goes for when I try to say something nice to myself too. It's easy for me to be nice to other people, and I'd much rather be helping someone else than letting someone help me, even Gil. I don't know why I'm like this, but I am."

Now it's your turn. What did you notice? Remember that the purpose of these activities is to help you listen to yourself with acceptance, understanding, compassion, and self-trust. Were you successful in doing that, or do you find criticism or self-blame, anger or frustration, impatience or demands to decide, change, or act in what you've just written? Can you reflect now with acceptance and compassion to help take the pressure off? Write your answers in your journal or use the form "Reflecting on Giving Myself Acceptance" at *www.guilford.com/zuckoff-forms*.

Self-Affirmation: Toward Self-Compassion and Self-Acceptance

Treating ourselves with compassion and viewing ourselves with acceptance can be especially challenging when we've been struggling with ambivalence. As we've seen, the reason is partly because we begin to blame ourselves for the trap we feel stuck in, growing increasingly frustrated and impatient with ourselves, and trying to push ourselves into action that we're not ready to take. The effect is to make us feel guilty, disgusted, or ashamed, and once those judgments take hold it's hard to escape the cycle of plummeting self-regard and increasing certainty that we'll never be able to get ourselves out of the mess we are in.

Self-acceptance and self-compassion are also made more difficult by many of the messages we receive on a daily basis from the world around us. We live in a critical culture. We're surrounded by advertisements that tell us all the ways in which we're lacking, so that we'll be motivated to buy the products that fill these gaps. People in authority often emphasize our shortcomings rather than our strengths when they evaluate us in the hope that this approach will motivate us to accomplish more. While criticism may have the intended effect of driving people to perform, it also leaves many of us more aware of what is wrong than of what is right with us.

Contrary to what many of us have come to believe, feeling genuinely good about ourselves promotes clarity of thought about the situations we are facing, hope for the future, and openness to positive change. And what helps us feel this way is focusing on and recognizing our own real and personally meaningful positive qualities, the essence of who we are, and allowing that recognition to inform how we see and think about ourselves. That's what the next group of activities is designed to help you do.

A list of "positive qualities you might possess" appears below. This list (adapted from one developed by motivational interviewing founders Bill Miller and Steve Rollnick[4]) was derived from experience with people who succeeded in making difficult decisions and positive changes in their lives. Read through the list and circle each word that names a quality you possess in some way (either here or in the form at *www.guilford.com/zuckoff-forms*). There's no "right" or "wrong" number, so don't worry if you're circling too many or too few. I've left some blanks at the bottom for you to add any qualities that I haven't listed.

- -
Positive Qualities You Might Possess

Accepting	Capable	Determined	Flexible
Active	Careful	Devoted	Focused
Adaptable	Caring	Discerning	Forgiving
Adventuresome	Charming	Disciplined	Friendly
Affectionate	Cheerful	Doer	Funny
Ambitious	Classy	Down-to-earth	Fun-loving
Appreciative	Clever	Driven	Generous
Articulate	Committed	Eager	Gentle
Artistic	Compassionate	Earnest	Gracious
Assertive	Confident	Easygoing	Grateful
Astute	Considerate	Efficient	Grounded
Athletic	Creative	Empathic	Handy
Attentive	Curious	Encouraging	Happy
Attractive	Cute	Energetic	Hardworking
Bold	Daring	Entertaining	Healthy
Brave	Decisive	Ethical	Helpful
Bright	Dedicated	Expressive	Honest
Calm	Deep	Faithful	Humble

---

[4]Miller, W. R., & Rollnick, S. (2013). *Motivational interviewing: Helping people change* (3rd ed., p. 218). New York: Guilford Press. Adapted by permission.

Imaginative	Passionate	Responsible	Sweet
Innocent	Patient	Savvy	Sympathetic
Insightful	Perceptive	Seductive	Tactful
Inspiring	Persistent	Self-aware	Tasteful
Intelligent	Playful	Selfless	Thorough
Interesting	Polite	Self-sufficient	Thoughtful
Introspective	Positive	Sensible	Tough
Kind	Powerful	Sensitive	Traditional
Lively	Practical	Sentimental	Trusting
Lovable	Prayerful	Serene	Trustworthy
Loving	Private	Sincere	Unconventional
Loyal	Prompt	Solid	Understanding
Mature	Protective	Spiritual	Upbeat
Meticulous	Questioning	Spontaneous	Virile
Modest	Quick	Stable	Visionary
Neat	Quiet	Steadfast	Vivacious
Nice	Realistic	Steady	Warm
Nonmaterialistic	Reasonable	Straightforward	Welcoming
Nurturing	Receptive	Streetwise	Well-read
Open	Reliable	Strong	Wise
Optimistic	Religious	Stubborn	Witty
Organized	Resourceful	Stylish	Worldly
Outgoing	Respectful	Supportive	Zestful

Now take a moment to reflect on completing this activity. What did you notice as you selected your positive qualities? Write your answers in your journal or in the form "Reflecting on Choosing My Positive Qualities" at *www.guilford.com/zuckoff-forms* after considering your companions' reflections on their choices:

- *Alec, who circled 84 qualities*: "I have a lot of good qualities. It made me think, 'My wife could be a lot worse off!' I'm not perfect or anything, but I work damn hard and am good at what I do. I did notice that most of these things show up either at work or at home—I don't do much that's outside those two places."

- *Barbara, who circled 56 qualities*: "I got stuck on some of these. Seeing 'passionate' made me think of who I used to be and how I want to be, but I know that's not who I am now. Seeing words like 'loyal' or 'devoted' was hard; I don't feel I have the right to describe myself in those ways because of the feelings I've been having. I guess it was hard not to focus on my problem during this exercise. But it was reassuring that there were quite a few positive qualities that I do feel I possess right now and that this whole thing hasn't completely blinded me to them."

- *Colin, who circled 95 qualities*: "I was surprised to find so many words to circle. I've always known I was different from other people, not just in my sexuality but in other ways. That's why I circled 'unconventional.' But it's a relief right now to see I also share a lot of qualities with other people because it makes me feel more normal. I added the word 'intense' because no other word quite describes my temperament. I noticed that I chose a lot of words that describe how I am in my relationship. I believe I possess those qualities, but this was hard to think about, given our current status."

- *Dana, who circled 68 qualities*: "At first I was noticing words I wished I could circle, like 'Happy,' or 'Calm,' or 'Optimistic.' I just don't think I am these things, not right now. That made me a little sad. But I didn't dwell on that, and I noticed that I had a lot of things to circle that I know are true about me, things that never change. That feels good."

- *Ellie, who circled 76 qualities*: "I have a lot more positive qualities than I thought, which is pretty nice to know. I liked that some qualities that I usually think are negative, like being quiet, which I often am in large groups, can be considered positive, which I guess it is at times (I'm a good listener). I must be lovable because my husband loves me and my children do, too. But I never really thought of it this way. I thought some of the words were funny. Are some people zestful? I guess they are. Not me, though."

Now look again at the words you circled and select the three that are the *most* characteristic of you. Then ask yourself what those words mean to you and why you chose them.

Your companions' answers appear below.

. . . .

The Positive Qualities
That Are Most Characteristic of Me

Alec

> **Hardworking, Helpful, Loyal**
>
> Hardworking and helpful: that's how I was raised—you do your work, the best that you're capable of, without complaining. And if you see someone who needs help, you offer it. That's what sales is all about, too—finding ways to help the customers and meet their needs. And being loyal goes along with that as well. I am loyal to my friends, my family, my employer, my customers, and I expect loyalty in return. If someone crosses me, he loses my loyalty. I expect a lot from people, and I think they have a right to expect a lot from me.

Barbara

> **Appreciative, Warm, Driven**
>
> My first thought was "How am I going to pick just three?" But when I looked them over these three jumped out at me. Appreciative is something that I feel about everything I have in my life. When I'm not feeling guilty and self-ish, I can genuinely have that feeling, and it shows. I have been told that I am a warm person. There's something about me that makes people gravitate toward me and feel good about themselves when they're around me. I like that quality very much. And driven—I sometimes feel as if there's a revving engine inside me that makes me want get things done. . . . I've always been that way. My parents told me that those "Energizer bunny" commercials reminded them of me when I was little. It certainly helped in raising my own three little go-go bunnies and handling all their activities.

Colin

> **Intense, Creative, Introspective—I want to add Loving, too**
>
> I know I'm a loving person, but it's hard to think about that right now. My intensity, creativity, and introspectiveness go together, so it's hard to sepa-rate them. I've always been very internal, very focused on my inner life and on trying to understand who I am and why I do what I do. It hasn't always been easy, but I wouldn't want to be any other way. It's the source of my creativity—I go inside, and ideas come to me. It can get very intense, but

without the intensity nothing interesting happens. I'm also intense in my relationships—I'm not someone who wants to have a lot of random people in my life, just a few who really mean something to me.

Dana

Stable, Sentimental, Gentle

Stable, grounded, solid—I don't seem to be rocked by things. I seem to have a core that remains the same; I don't fundamentally change who I am no matter what I go through. My friends and family can count on me to be there, and I can count on myself. I chose sentimental because that's something about me that I like but some people think is a little sappy. I don't show that side of myself to people who are not close to me. I get emotional when people express tender feelings toward each other, especially about special times in their past. And gentle pretty much means to me what it says—I try not to be harsh or careless with people, animals, or whatever.

Ellie

Devoted, Hardworking, Grateful, Strong, Generous, and Understanding

I couldn't narrow it down to just three. My family is the center of my life. I am very devoted to them, and I am extremely grateful to be blessed with them. I also think I am very hardworking at my job and in my home. I was raised to be that way. I hesitated writing down "strong" because I obviously don't have the strength to solve this weight problem, but I believe I'm strong in other ways. I have the strength to be there for others whenever they need to lean on me. And I think I am both generous and understanding. I would much rather give to others than receive, and I always seem to be able to understand people, and I try to show that understanding. I feel sort of conceited writing this down. I know I'm following the directions, but it does make me uncomfortable to say so many nice things about myself.

Now it's your turn. Ask yourself what each of the three words you chose means to you and why you picked those three, writing your answers in your journal or using the form at *www.guilford.com/zuckoff-forms*.

Now, as the last step in this activity, please select two of those three characteristics and recall a time when each of them showed itself especially clearly, describing the situation and how the characteristic revealed itself. First review your companions' responses on the following pages.

When Two of My Positive Qualities Showed Themselves

Alec

Loyal

My younger brother and his wife started having marital problems. There were times when I got angry with my brother because I knew that he was not innocent. But finally he called me one night, and he was almost crying. He said she had witnesses who saw him with another woman and that she was filing for divorce and she was going to make sure he never saw their kids again. I told him to come and stay with us until he was on his feet, and that I would pay for the best divorce attorney out there, and that he didn't need to worry about her threats. I think he must've told her I said those things because they ended up working out a custody agreement. He did stay with us for a while, and was really appreciative, and my wife backed me through all of that. She respects my loyalty to my family, and she knows I'd back her that way with her family members, too.

Helpful

One time that stands out was when my daughter was little and my mother-in-law was in the hospital. My wife was trying to juggle being with her mom and being with Jen, because she was at that stage where it was "mommy, mommy, mommy . . ." I was trying to be as available as possible for Jen, but that was tough because she wasn't as cooperative with me. So one night, Wendy was so exhausted, and she could see that Jen needed to spend some time with her. She just wanted to stay at home with her and rest, but she was afraid that no one would be there when the doctor came in to give a report on her mother's condition. Even though I was pretty tired myself, I went to the hospital and sat with her mother for the whole evening. We watched TV, talked, and when the doctor came in, I talked with him and put my wife on the phone, too. It just seemed like the right thing for me to do.

Barbara

Warm

My middle son was about 9 or 10 and at summer camp and I was working in the camp office. One night, one of the boys in his cabin came down with terrible pains in his abdomen. Everyone was very worried as they took the boy out of camp to the nearest hospital. Well, no one was going to sleep after that, and my son found his way over to the staff cabin to be near me. It wasn't long before his whole cabin was in my cabin, sleeping bags and all. Then several of the counselors showed up, and within an hour or so, I was completely surrounded. They spent the night telling stories and listening to music. It seemed as if they almost forgot what was happening once they came into my room. And the funniest part was that I was barely doing anything but sitting there! It was like they all gathered around me, felt better, and entertained each other. By morning, most of us had found a place to fall asleep, and we learned when we awoke that the boy was fine after having an appendectomy.

Driven

When I first became the coach of my daughter's volleyball team, I knew next to nothing about the sport, let alone how to coach it! But I could see that these girls needed help. The part-time coach they had was clearly not interested in continuing, and his attitude was atrocious. Long story short, within a few months, I had learned everything I could about the game and about coaching this age group. I studied, observed, and built positive relationships with all the girls. We practiced, practiced, practiced. We had fund-raisers and raised enough money to buy equipment plus new uniforms. I eventually got another very enthusiastic mother to assistant-coach, and together we helped that team get to the semifinals for the first time ever. We even had two of our players go on to play for the all-star team. Their parents were so proud and grateful. And the great thing is that the team continued to thrive even after we left the school. I sometimes take a little bit of pride in that, even though I'm no longer there.

Colin

Creative

When Paul and I were first together, we hung out at this club and had become fairly tight with a lot of the people there. Every year, they'd have a fantastic Halloween celebration, and everyone would try to outdo the costumes from the year before. I always designed and made ours. I enjoy the challenge, the intense focus on getting them perfect, and I particularly loved seeing Paul's admiring looks toward me as he watched each costume come together. He was always amazed at what I could do, and it made me feel like I was some sort of magician. We always got a lot of attention for my creations, and the year that we won first prize was pretty great. I remember him looking so happy that night. For me, though, the high point was him looking at me with that look of wonder and love. When we would look at each other that way, it felt like no one else was there or nothing else mattered.

Loving

I realize I want to write about being loving because it's important to me. Before we moved in together, Paul had this German shepherd, Annie. He loved that dog more than I'd ever seen someone love a pet. It endeared him to me right away. He spoke to her in such gentle tones, and she responded to his every mood and movement. Well, she came down with a disease that the vet said was only going to lead to suffering, so Paul made the decision to put her down. I went with him that night. I watched him carry her in, wrapped in her special afghan, and I marveled at how brave he was. When he came out alone, we drove to his place in silence. We had a drink, still in silence, and then he asked me if I'd stay. Then he curled up next to me and laid his head in my lap. I looked down at his face and saw a tear rolling down his cheek, then another. His tears turned to sobs, then they stopped and he fell asleep in my lap. I sat and held him for the rest of the night. I knew then that I would love him for the rest of my life. Later I made a piece for him—a painting/collage of him and Annie. It is still hanging in the room where she slept.

Dana

Sentimental

When I was a freshman in college, the girls from my floor had a movie night and watched Sleepless in Seattle. My roommate saw that I was crying quietly during the Empire State Building scene and acted really concerned about me. When I told her that I always cry in movies like that she busted out laughing. She thought something bad had happened to me that day. I told her I was just trying to hide my crying from the other girls. My family teases me about this, but I wasn't ready for teasing from these girls. After that, my roommate really changed toward me. I think she'd thought I was stuck up or aloof, and it turned out that other girls had a similar impression. My roommate started to say things like "Why don't we watch Sleepless again so we can all see Dana cry?" It was affectionate and actually made me feel good. Eventually, it became a thing—who could pick a movie that would make me cry. And I saw that I wasn't the only one. It was pretty funny, and we all bonded so tightly that year, and it all started with my stifled sobs! Now, when I see Sleepless, I feel sentimental about our dorm as well as the Empire State Building!

Stable

My cousin Karen died suddenly from an aneurysm when I was in high school. She was like a big sister to me. Her family lived on our street, and I spent so much time over there, she practically raised me. When she passed, it was a shock to everyone. At first, everyone was worried about how I was going to deal with her death. But that changed because I seemed to be dealing better than they were. I was hurting, I cried, I had some difficult times at school. But something inside me seemed to help me maintain my stability. I felt like I stayed who I was and felt heartbroken. I remember telling my mom that I was afraid of what life was going to feel like without Karen in it, but I guess I just accepted that that's the way it was. My friends sometimes tell me that

I'm like their "rock." I know they don't mean that I'm unfeeling; they just mean that I'm there if they need me, and I don't fall apart when they talk to me about their problems or when I have problems of my own.

Ellie

Devoted

I remember one Christmas Eve when my husband and I were up very late wrapping presents for the kids to put under the tree from Santa. I was coming down with the flu but didn't know it. Anyway, as I was putting the final touches on the packages, I felt this warmth come over me. It could've been a fever, but I said to my husband, "I don't think it gets any better than this." The next morning, I was sick as a dog, but when I saw the kids' faces— Theresa was only 2 at the time, she looked at the tree and gasped, literally with her mouth wide open, and said, "Momma, look, the Santa came to our house . . ." I started to cry, and I told my husband I was wrong the night before; this was the very best. I barely noticed how sick I was. Being devoted to them has given me so many gifts. I am so grateful for those memories.

Generous

I mostly think about being generous with my time, which is always in short supply. My niece called recently, and she was crying that she and her boyfriend broke up after she found out he'd been cheating. She asked if she could come over and talk since her parents were away. I had other plans that day, but I said yes. Well, she came over and talked and cried, and I tried to help, but it seemed like she needed more. So I asked my husband if we could take a rain check on the movie we'd planned to see, and he was fine with that. She spent the evening with us and then spent the night. It didn't take her hurt away, but I think it made her realize that she doesn't ever have to feel all alone, especially not when she was feeling that bad.

Now it's your turn. Please ask yourself: "What was the situation? How did the characteristic show itself?" Enter your answers in your journal or in the form at *www.guilford.com/zuckoff-forms*.

What feelings are you having now that you've reflected on your positive qualities? How are you seeing yourself right now? Write your answers to these questions in your journal or use the form "Reflecting on My Most Characteristic Positive Qualities" at *www.guilford.com/zuckoff-forms* after you consider your companions' reflections:

- *Alec:* "I'm feeling pretty good about myself, but I miss me and my wife being like we were. It seemed like back then she was on board with me more often and I felt good about doing things for her. I don't like to think about how long it's been since I felt that way. I felt more appreciated by her then. Remembering those times helps me realize I'm not just a guy who's always letting down his wife, and she's not a wife who just complains constantly. We can be good together."

- *Barbara*: "I am feeling happy, nostalgic, proud, bittersweet, and filled with appreciation for the memories I have with my children. I love thinking back on those times, but I think I miss it all so much that I try to put it out of my mind. How am I seeing myself? I loved and enjoyed my kids, and they had opportunities to enjoy me, but I also think I was a good role model. I showed them how to be an adult— to find a purpose and pursue it with everything you have and have fun while you're doing it!"

- *Colin*: "I definitely feel love for Paul and a longing for how things were between us at the beginning. I feel angry about losing that— not necessarily at him or at myself—just that it happened. And I feel some guilt and sadness for my part of it. I'm also very clear that I want us to be together. As for how I see myself, I'm more aware of how my situation has been negatively affecting my view of myself. It feels good to know that I am capable of loving someone so fully and of giving pleasure and joy."

- *Dana*: "I'm having happy feelings mostly, except remembering that my cousin is gone. And confident when I think about my friends from college and how I was able to become part of that group and how they all accepted me—I just love them all so much! It feels good to think about those great times. I know that I have a lot going for me, but I think I forget that sometimes, or I take for granted the strengths that I have, which makes me feel like I don't have as many."

- *Ellie*: "I am feeling some warm, cozy feelings right now. It makes me so happy to remember when the kids were small. I am also feeling grateful—God has filled my life with love. Looking at myself? Well, I'm feeling proud of myself for the moment at least. I like that I can be generous with others and loving and understanding. It gives me so much fulfillment in return. I wish I always felt this way!"

After you write your response, please listen to yourself as you read it out loud and allow yourself to stay with the feelings or thoughts that arise.

THE WAY FORWARD

If you've reached this part of the book by reading your way through it and doing all the activities, congratulations! You've already made a significant commitment of time and emotional energy, and that bodes well for your success in resolving your ambivalence and moving forward in your life. (If you've gotten here by skimming ahead or skipping activities, you can still choose to go back and work your way forward if and when the time is right and it seems helpful.)

The purpose of these last two chapters has been to reduce the power of the terrible triad of anxiety, avoidance, and self-blame to interfere with your decision about what is best for you and whether or not to take action toward change. Having helped you, I hope, take the pressure off and increase the sense of acceptance and compassion you feel from others and yourself, it's now time to address your dilemma head on, with a renewed and constructive focus on exploring your ambivalence in such a way as to help you to resolve it and move forward.

Do You Want to Change? Can You Change?

First Interlude
The Language of Change

In the late 1960s a psychologist named Daryl J. Bem offered a surprising proposal about how we develop the attitudes we hold and how those attitudes shape our behavior. We don't look inward to discover what we believe or how we should act, Bem claimed; we observe how we act, and then we form or change our attitudes based on what those actions tell us about ourselves. So you don't decide to eat an apple because you know you like apples; rather, if you eat an apple when given the chance, you decide you must like apples, or why else would you have eaten one?

This may strike you as an odd idea, and I surely don't think it captures the whole story of how people make decisions or choose what actions to take. Yet there is a kernel of truth to Bem's *self-perception theory*[1] that has important implications for our purpose here. That is, one way that we learn about ourselves is by paying attention to what we do—and, in particular, by listening to what we say when we talk about ourselves.

Almost everyone has had some experience with this. You start talking to your friend about a topic that's in the news—a political issue or something that happened on your favorite TV show. You think you're just making conversation . . . and before you know it you're getting pretty worked up, surprising your friend and yourself. When this happens, you might think, "I didn't realize how strongly I felt about this." Or you agree to do something you're not too sure you like, find yourself having a great time (or a lousy one), and suddenly realize, "Hey, I *like* (or, Whoa, I *hate*) this!"

---

[1]Bem, D. J. (1972). Self-perception theory. In L. Berkowitz (Ed.), *Advances in experimental social psychology* (Vol. 6, pp. 1–62). New York: Academic Press.

It's even possible that by now an experience like this has happened as you've completed the activities in this book. Like Alec becoming aware that his wife's doubts and mistrust bother him more than he'd recognized . . . Barbara's startled realization of how harshly she's been treating herself . . . Colin's surprise at the strength of his feelings when recalling events from decades earlier . . . Dana recognizing that telling herself there's no decision to make hasn't stopped her from facing a decision . . . Ellie noticing how she pushes away compliments and support even though she wishes for them. Through the process of writing out your own thoughts you, too, might already have learned something about yourself that you didn't know in quite that way before.

> We learn what we think as we hear ourselves speak.

Many approaches to counseling have recognized the value of inviting people to talk or write about their situation to help them "think out loud" about the choices they're facing. But the most truly innovative aspect of motivational interviewing lies in its recognition that how ready, willing, and able we become to change is strongly influenced by what we hear ourselves saying, to ourselves and to others, about the dilemma we face. When it comes to resolving ambivalence, the secret is to speak or write about the decision we're trying to make in a particular way, and to listen to ourselves in the right way, so that we can learn from ourselves what is best for us.

LISTENING WITH "EARS" TO OUR TALK ABOUT CHANGE

When we speak and write about the possibility of change, what should we be talking about? What should we be listening for and how should we be listening, if we're going to extricate ourselves from our dilemmas?

Research on the language of change has identified two complementary kinds of talk: *change talk*, or talk in favor of change, and *sustain talk*, or talk in favor of keeping things the way they are, of "sustaining" the status quo. Each of these kinds of talk, in turn, falls into two broad categories: *preparatory* talk and *mobilizing* talk. Preparatory talk includes expressions of:

- *Desire* to change ("I want to reduce my spending," "I wish I were more outgoing") or to stay the same ("I have no desire to exercise more," "I don't want to eat tasteless food just because it's healthier").

- *Ability* to change ("I could procrastinate less if I put my mind to it," "I know I can change my diet") or inability to change ("I can't quit smoking; it's too hard," "I don't think it's possible for me to lose weight").

- *Reasons* to change ("If I exercised, I'd have more energy," "I should try to socialize more, because I'd feel less lonely") or to stay the same ("Shopping is how I relax," "If I drank less, I would be more tense").
- *Need* to change ("I have to quit smoking," "I could die if I don't get control over my blood pressure") or to stay the same ("If I didn't have my private time, I'd go crazy," "I need my pain pills").

Mobilizing talk includes expressions of:

- *Commitment* to change ("I am going to start being nicer to myself," "I promise to stop cheating on you") or to stay the same ("I am going to keep gambling, and no one can stop me," "I will not change what I eat").
- *Activation* to change ("I'm ready to start looking for a new job," "I'm willing to try to control my anger") or to stay the same ("I'm prepared to accept a life without close relationships," "I'm not ready to forgive him for what he did").
- *Taking steps* to change ("I've begun to cut back on my drinking," "I ordered a blood glucose monitor so I can check my sugar") or to stay the same ("I canceled my appointment with the tutor," "I threw away my prescription").

What's the difference between preparatory talk and mobilizing talk? Imagine that you're standing with your fiancé in front of a judge or member of the clergy, who turns to you and asks: "Will you take this person to be your lawfully wedded spouse?" Now imagine that you respond, "I want to" or "I could" or "I have good reasons to" or "I need to." How well do you think that would go over with your beloved?[2]

Any response other than "I will!" is, of course, likely to get you in a lot of trouble. When you're asked for a promise, preparatory talk will not suffice. But how did you get to be standing there in the first place, ready to make the commitment your beloved is expecting? Through all the times you said to each other, "I want to be with you . . . We can make this work . . . We will be so happy . . . I have to have you in my life. . . ."

[2]Moyers, T. (2014). Do you swear? Motivational interviewing training new trainers manual (p. 173). Retrieved from *www.motivationalinterviewing.org/sites/default/files/tnt_manual_2014_d10_20150205.pdf.*

While mobilizing change talk expresses an intention to act, preparatory talk is all about preparing to make a decision or take action. Remember: Self-perception theory teaches us that we're not just saying what we already know when we talk this way; we're actually discovering our own attitudes and wishes as we listen to ourselves. Preparatory talk helps prepare us to make a decision about changing or remaining the same by shaping and clarifying our own attitudes about the issue or situation we are dealing with.

When people are ambivalent, their speech most commonly includes a mixture of preparatory change talk and preparatory sustain talk: "I know I should do this [*change talk*], but I'm worried about how it's going to affect me [*sustain talk*]. I've never tried anything like this before, and it might make things worse [*sustain talk*]. Besides, I'm not even sure I can do it [*sustain talk*]. The time is right to try, though [*change talk*], and when I think of how great I would feel if it goes well I get excited [*change talk*]. Still, I know it would be uncomfortable at first [*sustain talk*], and I don't know if it's worth doing that to myself [*sustain talk*]. But it might make things better in the long run [*change talk*]."

> Taking turns talking yourself into and out of change keeps you right where you are.

As you read these examples, did you feel as though you were being pulled one way and then the other, ending up no further along than where you started? This is what often happens when people talk to themselves when they're stuck in ambivalence: they end up going in circles. So I'm not going to invite you to listen to yourself switching back and forth between change talk and sustain talk, because you would literally be taking turns talking yourself into and out of change—with exactly the result you would expect. Instead, I'm going to help you *separate* the change talk from the sustain talk and explore your thoughts about change in a systematic way.

So that's my answer to the question of what we should be talking about and what we should be listening for if we want to help ourselves get unstuck. *How* should we be listening? It won't surprise you that my answer centers on self-acceptance and self-compassion. It's crucial that the work you've done to set aside judgment and control when thinking about your dilemma continues to guide you in the work ahead. My goal will be to help you listen to yourself with kindness and self-care, understand your own wishes and concerns more deeply, value your own thoughts and feelings, and trust yourself to make the decisions that are right for you.

How can I help you listen to yourself this way? I'm going to show you how to listen to yourself with "EARS":

- *Elaborate* further, by providing more descriptions and details as well as examples of what you've written about.
- *Affirm* your own values and goals as well as your own solutions to your dilemma.
- *Reflect* on what you've written, by highlighting the parts that stand out to you and thinking more about what they mean.
- *Summarize* your responses, by pulling together key thoughts and feelings so they can guide you in the direction that is best for you.

Listening to yourself with self-accepting EARS—without self-criticism or impatience—will help you write about your situation in the focused way that facilitates resolution of ambivalence.

IMPORTANCE OR CONFIDENCE: WHICH TO EXPLORE FIRST?

Until it becomes *important* to you to change and you become *confident* that you can succeed, readiness to commit to a clear direction will remain elusive. Each of these dimensions of motivation requires separate attention, and rating yourself on importance and confidence again can help you decide which pathway will be most useful to follow from here.

First, let's look at your companions' new self-ratings on these dimensions and their thoughts about why they chose the numbers they did.

Importance and Confidence for the First Interlude

How **important** is it to me *right now* to make the change I am considering?

0	I	2	3	4	5	6	7	8	9	10

Not at all   Moderately   Extremely

How **confident** am I *right now* that I would be able to make that change?

0	I	2	3	4	5	6	7	8	9	10

Not at all   Moderately   Extremely

Alec, who initially gave himself a 3 for importance and a 9 for confidence, now gives himself a **4** and a **5**:

> "I'm not so mad at my wife now. I still don't like her nagging, but I can see more where she's coming from, missing me and how we were. And I have to admit there's a couple of things going on that I'm not happy about. I still think my doctor went too far, but my buddy telling me about his heart thing did shake me a little. And not applying for the promotion—maybe I'm not so sure I want to ratchet up my time commitment at work even more right now, which is what it would take. But I'm too young to settle for what I have now. All in all, the drinking doesn't seem the most important part of what's going on. And trying to change that would complicate my life at work. I'm not sure I want to do anything about it even though maybe there's room for improvement, and honestly doing something about it wouldn't be that easy."

Barbara, who initially gave herself a 5 for importance and a 2 for confidence, now gives herself a **6** and a **4**:

> "It's so painful for me to think about what it would do to Steve if I were to tell him I want something different, I haven't even let myself think about why I've been feeling the way I am. I can see now that's never going to work. I can't stay with Steve out of guilt and fear and shame when I want so much more. But I can't decide right now to leave, either. I really don't have any idea what's going on with me, so I need to give myself time to look at why I'm having these intense urges and what my options are. Without putting 'pressure' on myself, right? So 6 because I know I have to go about making this decision in a different way from how I've made decisions in the past. And 4 because doing these activities has helped me remember what I'm capable of, and I think if I trust myself a little more I'm going to be able to figure it out."

Colin, who initially gave himself an 8 for importance and a 7 for confidence, now gives himself a **5** and a **5**:

> "Maybe I should want to do something about my anger just because it upsets Paul. But obviously I'm more conflicted than I thought when I started this, and if I'm going to change who I am, the reason has to come from me. I learned that a long time ago, but it seems I needed

to remember it. So I've got to make sense of how I feel, for both of our sakes. And that's where the confusion comes in. I can't pretend that how I express anger is completely okay, but I'm not sure how bad it is. I know I'm not a bad person and I have to be able to stand up for myself. It's time for me to look at *all this* more closely before I put any more focus on making myself change. Maybe if I were sure about what I want to do, it wouldn't be so hard for me to do it."

Dana, who initially gave herself a 6 for importance and a 4 for confidence, now gives herself an **8** and a **6**:

"Ever since I can remember I've been telling myself to make mature choices about what to do with my life. But is it mature to do what your parents and your family think is right when it's not what you really want? I want to teach. I should stop trying to convince myself that's not how I feel and start taking myself seriously. So that's why I chose an 8 for importance. But I chose a 6 for confidence because it's still kind of scary to think about doing something risky. I can't really blame my parents for that; I do think about what they would say, but I'm the one who worries about how things will turn out for me if I do something impractical. And it's understandable that I'm scared. But I also know that I'm strong and stable and have a lot going for me and that's why I'm feeling a little more confident."

Ellie, who initially gave herself a 10 for importance and a 0 for confidence, now gives herself an **8** and a **2**:

"I'm never really going to accept being overweight. The only things that are really a 10 to me are my kids and my husband—but getting this weight off is definitely next in line. I'd be lying if I said knew how, but I do feel different, and I did realize a couple of things. One is that I'm mixed up about taking care of everybody all the time. Something's not right when you spend half your time wishing someone would share the work and the other half telling people you don't need any help. Maybe I don't want help, but why the heck not? The other thing is that I need to stop these mental beatings I give myself about dieting and eating. It's bad enough feeling fat and self-conscious and knowing that other people are probably thinking not so nice things about you. Piling more abuse on yourself only makes things worse. I've got to start reminding myself about the good things about me, like I did in the last chapter."

Reassessing Importance and Confidence: Your Turn

Now it's time to rate yourself again on the same scale. Please circle the number that best captures where you are in terms of the importance of making the change you've been considering and your confidence that you could succeed if you decided to do it. Use the rating scale on page 89 or the form "Importance and Confidence for the First Interlude" at *www.guilford.com/zuckoff-forms*. In your journal or the form "Importance and Confidence for the First Interlude," write down your thoughts about why you chose the numbers you did.

THE WAY FORWARD

Should your next step be Chapter 4 or Chapter 5? In general, if you're undecided about whether you want, need, or have good reasons to change, it will be most helpful to begin by exploring the importance of change to you; if you feel certain about your decision, but pessimistic that you will be able to succeed in carrying it out, it will be more helpful to begin by exploring and strengthening your confidence for change. However, if your confidence is low enough, it can create doubt about whether you've made the right decision, and if importance is low enough, it can undermine your confidence. I address these complexities in the next two chapters, but for now, here are my recommendations for where to go next:

- Importance = 0? Chapter 4
- Importance = 1–5? Chapter 4 (unless Confidence = 0, then Chapter 5)
- Importance = 6–7? Chapter 4 (unless Confidence = 0–2, then Chapter 5)
- Importance = 8? Chapter 4 (unless Confidence = 0–4, then Chapter 5)
- Importance = 9–10? Chapter 5 (unless Confidence = 7–10, then Chapter 4)

Following these recommendations, Alec, Barbara, Colin, and Dana will all go directly to Chapter 4 and then on to Chapter 5; Ellie, whose importance for change is high but whose confidence for change is low, will complete Chapter 5 first and then return to complete Chapter 4. Once you've decided on your next step, let's continue.

• • • • 4 • • • •

Exploring the Importance of Change to You

When it comes to resolving ambivalence, I've said that half the battle is finding a way forward whose benefits or advantages dramatically outweigh its costs or disadvantages for you. (The other half—believing you can succeed at getting where you want to go—is the focus of Chapter 5.) However, choosing a direction is not a simple matter of "adding up" a list of pros and cons; if it were, no one would stay stuck for very long. Various advantages or disadvantages can carry more or less "weight," depending on what matters most to you and the feelings you experience when you consider your options. Some of the benefits of change may not be obvious at first, and sometimes what you might have to give up to pursue a new and unknown path can scare you away from even considering the possibility seriously. So, as I wrote in Chapter 1, resolving ambivalence requires untangling the complicated and conflicting thoughts you have about the issue you're struggling with while allowing your feelings about it to inform, but not overwhelm, your decision on the direction that's right for you.

To begin the exploration of your thoughts and feelings about the importance of change, I'd like you to ask yourself why you chose that number for the importance of change on page 89 and not a *lower* number. (If you chose 2, why didn't you choose 0? If you chose 5, why not 1 or 2? If you chose 8, why not just 3 or 4?) But first, consider your companions' responses, shown on pages 94 and 95.

Why Did I Choose That Number Rather Than a Lower One?

Alec

Importance = 4

> When we're out with friends, I don't even drink that much, so this has nothing to do with me having a "drinking problem." (Not that we've seen our friends all that often lately because of how many hours I work, which is not too great.) It bothers my wife that drinking is part of my work life, and I don't like how things have gotten between us. My life would be easier if there wasn't so much tension at home. Also I don't want to wait until something happens to me and some doctor says I have to quit. Alcohol relaxes me, and I enjoy it. And I'm not going to let my future pass me by, and that's what would happen if suddenly I couldn't take my customers out for drinks. Wendy needs to appreciate that and not try to control my decisions.

Barbara

Importance = 6

> I need to be fulfilled in my life. I can't be satisfied with "settling." I have to have challenges to meet. I need excitement—that scared, exhilarated feeling when you're not sure you can handle something but you're going to do it anyway. But just writing these things makes me feel scared and guilty. It's a struggle not to start talking myself out of it. I've spent almost 30 years devoting myself to taking care of the people I love and doing one hell of a job at it, too. How could I throw that all away? So it's important for me to leave, and it's important for me to stay. Okay, I'm not going to talk myself out of my own feelings. What's really important is for me to pay attention to them in a serious way. It's not normal for me not to know what I want, but that's where I am, and it's a step forward to say that. I am a person who deals with problems head on. So that's what I need to do now.

Colin

Importance = 5

> To be quite honest, I put a 5 because I couldn't put a higher number. I don't want to hurt Paul. I don't want to lose him. But this issue is starting to rub up against something else in me. I don't want to have to give up things that are important to me, like my integrity, like the ability to keep people from getting over on me or treating me disrespectfully. And I don't want to have to be the bad guy in the relationship, because that's not fair to me. I can't tell whether this is my pride, my stubbornness, or some acquired wisdom on my part. All I know is that I'm not so ready anymore to agree with this idea

> that I just need to change and everything will work out. That hasn't been working for me anyway.

Dana

Importance = 8

> I know that I want to teach. I know that I am happy and feel fulfilled when I am working with children. I want to have that feeling again of waking up excited to face the day. I used to feel that way at my job. But I haven't felt that way for a while now, and I'm pretty sure that feeling isn't coming back if I stay where I am. I guess I've been feeling as if my life has been on hold, and I've been trying to talk myself into seeing it as not so bad. But I have to do something with my life where I feel like I'm making a difference in someone else's life, and I know I could do that as a teacher. That doesn't mean that I'm still not worried about taking the plunge, because I am. It's just that I can feel now how much it matters to me.

Ellie

Importance = 8

> My weight casts a shadow over almost everything in my life. Trying to ignore it has made me feel even worse inside. I walk into a room and the first thing I do is check out the size of any female person around my age. I get so self-conscious when there's food around that I try not to eat, and if I do, I'm wondering what people are thinking about me. When Gil tries to be affectionate, I don't even want him to touch me. If I could lose weight, I honestly feel like I'd become almost a different person. I could feel more relaxed, even when I'm alone. I could get excited about going clothes shopping for the first time in ages. I could look forward to events without stressing over what I'll wear and what I'll look like. I'd be able to socialize with family and friends without feeling so down or uptight.

Now it's your turn. Please ask yourself: "Why did I choose that number for the importance of change and not a number that was 2, 3, or 4 *lower*?" That is, "What makes the change I'm considering as important as it is to me right now?" Enter your responses in your journal or use the form at *www.guilford.com/zuckoff-forms*.

Change Talk or Sustain Talk?

Next I'd like you to mark all the instances of change talk and all the instances of sustain talk in your response. To help you recognize the two types of talk, the responses of your companions are shown below with change talk highlighted and sustain talk underlined.

Why Did I Choose That Number Rather Than a Lower One?

Alec

Importance = 4

When we're out with friends, I don't even drink that much, so this has nothing to do with me having a "drinking problem." (Not that we've seen our friends all that often lately because of how many hours I work, which is not too great.) It bothers my wife that drinking is part of my work life, and I don't like how things have gotten between us. My life would be easier if there wasn't so much tension at home. Also I don't want to wait until something happens to me and some doctor says I have to quit. Alcohol relaxes me, and I enjoy it. And I'm not going to let my future pass me by, and that's what would happen if suddenly I couldn't take my customers out for drinks. Wendy needs to appreciate that and not try to control my decisions.

Barbara

Importance = 6

I need to be fulfilled in my life. I can't be satisfied with "settling." I have to have challenges to meet. I need excitement—that scared, exhilarated feeling when you're not sure you can handle something but you're going to do it anyway. But just writing these things makes me feel scared and guilty. It's a struggle not to start talking myself out of it. I've spent almost 30 years devoting myself to taking care of the people I love and doing one hell of a job at it, too. How could I throw that all away? So it's important for me to leave, and it's important for me to stay. Okay, I'm not going to talk myself out of my own feelings. What's really important is for me to pay attention to them in a serious way. It's not normal for me not to know what I want, but that's where I am, and it's a step forward to say that. I am a person who deals with problems head on. So that's what I need to do now.

Colin

Importance = 5

To be quite honest, I put a 5 because I couldn't put a higher number. I don't want to hurt Paul. I don't want to lose him. But this issue is starting to rub up against something else in me. I don't want to have to give up things that are important to me, like my integrity, like the ability to keep people from getting over on me or treating me disrespectfully. And I don't want to have to be the bad guy in the relationship, because that's not fair to me. I can't tell whether this is my pride, my stubbornness, or some acquired wisdom on my part. All I know is that I'm not so ready anymore to agree with this idea that I just need to change and everything will work out. That hasn't been working for me anyway.

Dana

Importance = 8

I know that I want to teach. I know that I am happy and feel fulfilled when I am working with children. I want to have that feeling again of waking up excited to face the day. I used to feel that way at my job. But I haven't felt that way for a while now, and I'm pretty sure that feeling isn't coming back if I stay where I am. I guess I've been feeling as if my life has been on hold, and I've been trying to talk myself into seeing it as not so bad. But I have to do something with my life where I feel like I'm making a difference in someone else's life, and I know I could do that as a teacher. That doesn't mean that I'm still not worried about taking the plunge, because I am. It's just that I can feel now how much it matters to me.

Ellie

Importance = 8

My weight casts a shadow over almost everything in my life. Trying to ignore it has made me feel even worse inside. I walk into a room and the first thing I do is check out the size of any female person around my age. I get so self-conscious when there's food around that I try not to eat, and if I do, I'm wondering what people are thinking about me. When Gil tries to be affectionate, I don't even want him to touch me. If I could lose weight, I honestly feel like I'd become almost a different person. I could feel more relaxed, even when I'm alone. I could get excited about going clothes shopping for the first time in ages. I could look forward to events without stressing over what I'll wear and what I'll look like. I'd be able to socialize with family and friends without feeling so down or uptight.

Now it's your turn. Please mark all the instances of change talk and all the instances of sustain talk in your response. If you're not sure whether something you wrote is change talk or sustain talk, leave it unmarked; if you think it might be both, mark it as both. If you're highlighting (either in your journal entry or in the online form), use different colors so you can easily identify the two kinds of talk. If you're using pencil or pen, circle the change talk and underline the sustain talk.

Just like your companions, it's likely that your response included both change talk and sustain talk. To help you reduce the flipping back and forth that keeps you stuck, I need to help you identify which side of your ambivalence to focus on now. The answer lies in the balance between change talk and sustain talk.

If you found more change talk than sustain talk, whether the balance is weighted heavily (as it is for Dana and Ellie) or more lightly (as it is for Barbara), skip the next section and go on to the following one, "Exploring the Importance of Change" (p. 103). If the balance is even, as it is for Alec, I'd also recommend that you skip the next section, at least for now. (You can always come back to it later if becomes important to do so.) However, if you found the balance weighted clearly toward sustain talk, like Colin, then please continue to the next section, "Exploring the Importance of the Status Quo," where I will first invite you to take a closer look at your personal importance for staying the same. And, if you found a good deal of change talk, but nonetheless feel as though it would be valuable for you to take some time to explore the "status quo" side of your ambivalence, you are of course welcome to continue to the next section as well. As always, you are the best judge of what will be helpful for you.

EXPLORING THE IMPORTANCE
OF THE STATUS QUO

When I invited you to think about why the change you've been considering is as important to you as it is right now, you found yourself thinking about your desire, reasons, or need not to change. Why?

One reason that might have happened is actually related more to confidence than to importance. When people have significant doubts about whether it would be possible to accomplish a goal, those doubts can "bleed over" and affect their sense of the importance of change as well. After all, as I noted in Chapter 1, it's distressing to believe that you have a problem but there's nothing you can do about it, and one way people can protect themselves from those distressed feelings is by trying to minimize the seriousness of the problem or the need for change.

How can you tell whether this is a significant contributor to your attraction to maintaining the status quo? Imagine for a moment that you have come up with a plan for making the change you're considering that you are 100% certain would succeed. If your confidence for change were a 10, how important (on the 0–10 scale) would making the change be to you right now? If the number you chose is significantly higher than the one you chose at the end of the First Interlude, then please stop reading this chapter for now and go on to Chapter 5. Trying to resolve your ambivalence about the best direction for you with the nagging feeling that you are wasting your time because you won't be able to accomplish it anyway is likely to end in frustration and discouragement. After you have completed the activities designed to enhance your confidence in your ability to make the change you are considering, please come back to this chapter, starting with the next section, "Exploring the Importance of Change."

If your number for importance stayed the same, however, the reason almost certainly goes back to the core insight I cited in the Prelude as the starting point for this book: there are good reasons you haven't made the change you've been considering. As we saw in the case of Sheila, ignoring or minimizing those reasons when they come to the forefront of your mind won't make them go away; in fact, it's likely to make them assert themselves even more strongly. So your response to the question about the importance of change is a clear signal to think seriously about and honor your reasons for keeping things the way they are.

I'd like you to start with the reasons you've already written about. Please list each instance of sustain talk in your previous response. How you group or separate them is up to you; there's no right or wrong way, but you can emulate Colin's approach (shown below) by using the form at *www.guilford.com/zuckoff-forms*; otherwise use your own organization in your journal. What's important is to give meaningful consideration to each reason you have for preferring the status quo.

Once you've listed your reasons, please ask yourself these questions about each one:

- "What did I mean by this? How can I describe it more fully?"
- "What makes this reason important to me? What would happen if I disregard it?"

. . . .

Reasons for Keeping Things the Same

Colin

My integrity.

What did I mean by this? How can I describe it more fully?

I cannot "admit" that something is wrong that I don't really believe is wrong. I think that's what I was trying to make myself do, to allow my *judgment to be replaced by Paul's, instead of honestly looking at what I've been doing and arriving at my own decision.*

What makes this reason important to me? What would happen if I disregard it?

My integrity is all I have control over. If I give up being who I am, then who does Paul end up with anyway? So being true to myself is not only something I have to do for me, it's also what I need to do for him.

The ability to keep people from getting over on me or getting away with treating me disrespectfully.

What did I mean by this? How can I describe it more fully?

A long time ago I decided that I would not trust anyone but myself to look out for me. I kept my promise to myself that I'd never let anyone get away with pressuring me into doing something that didn't feel right. And I learned that getting angry can be a pretty effective way of doing that. Every time I stand up and someone who's been trying to take advantage of me backs down I feel stronger and more in control.

What makes this reason important to me? What would happen if I disregard it?

The world is full of people who don't care what they have to do to other people to get what they want. If there were more people like me, they wouldn't get away with so much. Disregard this? That would make me a victim in waiting. Too many people are too afraid to stand up. I feel bad for them. I'm not about to be one of them, and I like to believe that my refusing to back down might help to protect the scared ones, too.

I don't want to have to be the bad guy in the relationship, because that's not fair to me.

What did I mean by this? How can I describe it more fully?

I will admit that I cannot fully explain some of my own behavior. But I know that I am a good person and a loving partner. And that there have been plenty of times when I had a right to be angry with Paul. So the solution has to take into account Paul's contributions to the problems we've had as well as mine.

What makes this reason important to me? What would happen if I disregard it?

If I let myself be the "bad guy" without Paul understanding my feelings, how can I feel worth loving? How could I live with myself?

It's important, as you consider your reasons not to change, that you take the full picture into account; only then can you weigh these reasons meaningfully. It's also important to explore this side of the decisional balance thoroughly now, to prevent reasons or concerns you've neglected from coming up when I invite you explore your reasons for changing; we don't want to re-create the "I want to—I don't want to—I should—I shouldn't . . ." ambivalence circle that you've already had too much experience with and are trying to escape.

Often, when people start to explore the reasons they thought of, they find that other reasons begin to emerge as well. You may already have more "sustain talk" running through your mind than you've written about. On the other hand, sometimes those other reasons don't come to mind until someone asks us (or we ask ourselves), *"What else* do I think about this?"

So that's your next step: to ask yourself, "What else might make me feel that *not* making a change is the right decision for me? What are some other good things about the way things are, or the way I am, now? And what other disadvantages would there be of making a change? What else am I afraid of losing or having to give up?"

Consider Colin's responses, shown below, before you write your own in your journal or using the form at *www.guilford.com/zuckoff-forms.*

. . . .

More Reasons for Keeping Things the Same

Colin

What else makes not changing right for me? What else is good about the status quo?

> Paul and I are in a place where something finally has to give. Things have not been good between us for some time now and, although it makes me feel sad to write this, there's the possibility of relief in throwing in the towel. Maybe we should both find someone we're more compatible with. Starting to feel a little more like myself makes me wonder if letting it end would be for the best.

What other disadvantages would there be? What else am I afraid of having to give up?

> If I compromise myself to accommodate to Paul, I think I could lose my spontaneity, my passion—ironically, a lot of what attracted him to me in the first place. I don't want to be in a passionless relationship, and I'm afraid that's where we'll be headed if I try to do what he wants from me.

. . . .

Reflecting on the Importance of Keeping Things the Same

The purpose of the activities in this section was to invite you to honor and explore the reasons you have for keeping things the way they are rather than making a change. Please reread what you wrote in response to these two sets of questions and ask yourself: "Where does this leave me now? How am I feeling about keeping things the same?" Write your answers in your journal or use the form "Reflecting on the Importance of Keeping Things the Same" at *www.guilford.com/zuckoff-forms*. But consider Colin's reflections first:

> "These hopeless thoughts have been swimming around in the back of my mind for longer than I like to think about; I've just never let myself say them. But seeing them now, in black and white, all I can think is: What? Paul is the best thing that has ever happened to me. And I'm going to walk away because it hurts him when I yell at him and he wants me to stop doing that? Everything I think about a lot of people not caring about anyone but themselves or about how they hurt you might be true, but I've been acting like Paul is one of them! And that makes no sense at all. Maybe I had to come out and say the most extreme thing before I could truly know that it's not how I really feel. Maybe I just needed to know I could say it, not be afraid of it. All I know now is that this is not what I want. I do need to be able to maintain my integrity, and I do need to feel like I'm a not bad person. But I need to do those things with Paul, not without him. So, here's what I think now: I don't necessarily have to change how I do anger everywhere. And Paul is not perfect, and sometimes I am going to get mad at him. But not the way I've been doing it."

Sometimes, as Colin's response shows, reflecting on reasons not to change triggers thoughts about a desire, need, or reasons for change. To make sure any such thoughts are included, highlight any instances of change talk in your reflection and add them to your list.

Here's what Colin's reflection, with change talk highlighted, looks like:

> "These hopeless thoughts have been swimming around in the back of my mind for longer than I like to think about; I've just never let myself say them. But seeing them now, in black and white, all I can think is: What? Paul is the best thing that has ever happened to me.

And I'm going to walk away because it hurts him when I yell at him and he wants me to stop doing that? Everything I think about a lot of people not caring about anyone but themselves or about how they hurt you might be true, but I've been acting like Paul is one of them! And that makes no sense at all. Maybe I had to come out and say the most extreme thing before I could truly know that it's not how I really feel. Maybe I just needed to know I could say it, not be afraid of it. All I know now is that this is not what I want. I do need to be able to maintain my integrity, and I do need to feel like I'm a not bad person. But I need to do those things with Paul, not without him. So, here's what I think now: I don't necessarily have to change how I do anger everywhere. And Paul is not perfect, and sometimes I am going to get mad at him. But not the way I've been doing it."

EXPLORING THE IMPORTANCE OF CHANGE

Please list each of the instances of change talk in your response at the beginning of this chapter and in your reflection in the previous section, if you completed it. How you group or separate them is up to you; there's no right or wrong way. It's fine to break up sentences if different parts of a sentence mean different things to you. If you want to prepare a list the way your companions did (shown below), you can use the form at *www.guilford. com/zuckoff-forms*, or come up with your own approach for your journal. Then ask yourself these questions about each one:

- "What did I mean by this? What more can I say about it to describe it more fully?"
- "What makes this reason important to me? What would happen if I disregarded it?"

. . . .

Reasons for Change

Alec

When we're out with friends, I don't even drink that much.

What did I mean by this? How can I describe it more fully?

> I don't seem to feel the need to have more than a couple when I'm out with friends, as opposed to when I'm out with customers.

What makes this reason important to me? What would happen if I disregarded it?

> This isn't a reason for me to cut down—more like an interesting observation. Not sure what it means.

Not that we've seen our friends all that often lately because of how many hours I work, which is not too great.

What did I mean by this? How can I describe it more fully?

> It does seem like my life outside of work has decreased over the years, and it hasn't been too good for me or for my marriage. Hanging with friends was a stress reducer, plus it gave us time together doing something besides worrying about bills and taking care of Jen. On the way home we'd make fun of their crazy marriages, and they probably did the same thing about us. It was all good.

What makes this reason important to me? What would happen if I disregarded it?

> I guess I <u>have</u> been disregarding our life outside of work. We don't have much fun together. Maybe I've been forgetting why I bust my butt at work. Makes me wonder if we did start doing some things together if that could reduce some of the stress. I don't know how she'd feel about that, but having something to look forward to at the end of the week could be beneficial to my sanity.

It bothers my wife that drinking is part of my work life, and I don't like how things have gotten between us. My life would be easier if there wasn't so much tension at home.

What did I mean by this? How can I describe it more fully?

> I miss the good times with Wendy. Maybe if drinking wasn't such an issue, our relationship would've gone in a better direction. It's like a wedge between us.

What makes this reason important to me? What would happen if I disregarded it?

> I don't like how distant we are from each other and how strained it feels a lot of times. I get home, and she starts in on me about drinking and coming home late, and I come back at her, and then I go off by myself.

I don't want to wait until something happens to me and some doctor says I have to quit.

What did I mean by this? How can I describe it more fully?

> When Jim said his doctor told him to quit drinking, I could see that he was more freaked out by his doctor's advice than by the fibrillations. Which I

definitely get. So that makes me think it would be smart to cut back a little and drop a few pounds so nothing like that happens to me.

What makes this reason important to me? What would happen if I disregarded it?

I have to admit that it would be pretty stupid to just disregard this warning. It does seem logical to do something as long as it makes sense to me. I always believed that people should keep some sort of balance—you know, everything in moderation. I didn't really notice how things have gotten out of balance.

Barbara

I need to be fulfilled in my life.

What did I mean by this? How can I describe it more fully?

This sounds selfish to me, but I don't mean it in a selfish way. I need to be doing something that is meaningful to me. I was fulfilled being a mother, and that is far from a selfish role. But the kids no longer require me to be involved with their daily lives. That has left a hole, and nothing is there to fill it.

What makes this reason important to me? What would happen if I disregarded it?

I have to find a way to fill that hole. Disregarding this would leave me miserable and restless, as I've been. It's not an option to disregard this anymore.

I can't be satisfied with "settling."

What did I mean by this? How can I describe it more fully?

It is of no use for me to keep telling myself that I should try to be like some other women I see. I'm not saying that there's anything wrong with what those women want from life, but I cannot go on judging myself and saying that I want too much.

What makes this reason important to me? What would happen if I disregarded it?

I wouldn't feel alive. The thought of that feels not quite like death, but more like being an automaton, going through the motions of life until the end arrives. That's not for me. I'm not done yet.

I have to have challenges to meet.

What did I mean by this? How can I describe it more fully?

It's this intense desire to accomplish things, to feel like I have something to offer, that pushes me to grow and to develop my abilities further. This is not a selfish wish on my part—at least I don't see it that way now. I don't want more things; I want more life in my life.

What makes this reason important to me? What would happen if I disregarded it?

This is who I am. I cannot just make these feelings disappear as I've been trying to do.

I need excitement—that scared, exhilarated feeling when you're not sure you can handle something but you're going to do it anyway.

What did I mean by this? How can I describe it more fully?

This is how I felt when Joe asked me out for coffee. It felt, for just a moment, very exciting and full of possibilities. But if I let myself stay with that fantasy, it doesn't feel good. The excitement is gone when I envision it in reality. Well, that's a realization. I think I can honestly say that I don't want to act on that sort of urge with another man.

What makes this reason important to me? What would happen if I disregarded it?

I can't disregard this need for excitement any more than I can ignore the other needs I've been describing. They all go together, as I think about it, so it's not an option. But if I'm not going to find fulfillment in another man, I will have to find it somewhere else, and that's where I draw a blank. So there's a relief in this but also uncertainty and discomfort.

I'm not going to talk myself out of my own feelings. What's really important is for me to pay attention to them in a serious way. I am a person who deals with problems head on. So that's what I need to do now.

What did I mean by this? How can I describe it more fully?

This is what I'm doing, right here, for the first time. That's the part that feels good.

What makes this reason important to me? What would happen if I disregarded it?

Disregarding this is exactly what I've been doing; it's gotten me nowhere.

Colin

I don't want to hurt Paul. I don't want to lose him.

What did I mean by this? How can I describe it more fully?

It has never, ever been my intention to hurt him. When I think of how my life was before I met him, it doesn't even seem real. I've grown in ways that I never envisioned from how we've loved each other.

What makes this reason important to me? What would happen if I disregarded it?

> Losing Paul would mean losing the most important person in my life, and I can't let that happen.

Paul is the best thing that has ever happened to me. And I'm going to walk away because it hurts him when I yell at him and he wants me to stop doing that?

What did I mean by this? How can I describe it more fully?

> When I wrote this, I felt like someone was turning the lights back on in a room that I'd let fade into the dark. As complicated as this all seems to be, in a way it's really simple. Why would he stay with me if being with me makes him hurt? And what kind of person would I be if I'm not willing, really willing, to stop doing what hurts him?

What makes this reason important to me? What would happen if I disregarded it?

> Knowing what you really want is very clarifying. And disregarding it would be like betraying myself even more than betraying Paul.

But I've been acting like Paul is one of them! And that makes no sense at all.

What did I mean by this? How can I describe it more fully?

> Once I get angry I treat Paul like he's the enemy. I just see someone who wants to hurt me and doesn't care about me at all. So of course it feels like I'm trying to destroy him, because when I'm caught up in those feelings I probably am. But just because we're not on the same side when we argue doesn't mean I have to forget who he is and that he loves me.

What makes this reason important to me? What would happen if I disregarded it?

> I never thought about it this way before. This is probably the most important thing I've realized, and I need to let it sink in some more.

I do need to be able to maintain my integrity, and I do need to feel like I'm not a bad person. But I need to do those things with Paul, not without him. Sometimes I am going to get mad at him. But not the way I've been doing it.

What did I mean by this? How can I describe it more fully?

> I have to figure out how to have him and still be me. If I do get mad, I can't pretend I'm not. But I have to learn to get mad without overwhelming him. I also have to be able to admit my part of our problems without the story becoming "Colin was terrible, and now he's ashamed."

What makes this reason important to me? What would happen if I disregarded it?

> I don't have much leeway with Paul at this point, so I have to change how I express anger toward him. I'm not sure how. I don't think I can do it on my own. Maybe that's the problem—thinking I should be able to. I know I'm not answering the questions, but this feels more important. Maybe the point is that this is our problem and the only way we're going to solve it is together. That's worth thinking about more.

Dana

I know that I want to teach. I know that I am happy and feel fulfilled when I am working with children.

What did I mean by this? How can I describe it more fully?

> Even in college when I was telling myself to stop spending all that time figuring out things to do with the kids, I knew it was true, because it made me happier than anything. I just wouldn't let myself know I knew it.

What makes this reason important to me? What would happen if I disregarded it?

> That's what I've done until now: disregarded it. But I could never make it really go away even though I tried. Now I don't want to imagine spending the rest of my life doing something that doesn't make me happy.

I want to have that feeling again of waking up excited to face the day. I haven't felt that way for a while now, and I'm pretty sure that feeling isn't coming back if I stay where I am.

What did I mean by this? How can I describe it more fully?

> I am typically an enthusiastic person who welcomes each day. I had that feeling when I started at my job because it was exciting to earn money and handle responsibility. Nothing about this job gives me that feeling now. But I do get that feeling when I'm thinking about teaching.

What makes this reason important to me? What would happen if I disregarded it?

> I have actually been trying to "disregard" the absence of this feeling too, by telling myself that no job is satisfying all the time and that I have to be realistic about life. But that hasn't really worked either. Forcing myself to go day by day, trying to turn lemons into lemonade, isn't changing the way I feel.

I've been feeling as if my life has been on hold.

What did I mean by this? How can I describe it more fully?

> I feel like I've been waiting for something to get better. It's important to me that I didn't start looking for a way out as soon as the job got boring. And I didn't just complain. I worked to the best of my abilities to show them that I am a valuable, bright, motivated employee, but they still treat me like a gofer. And I tried to change my own attitude by focusing on positive aspects of the job. That didn't work either. There is truly no future for me there.

What makes this reason important to me? What would happen if I disregarded it?

> I'd just keep trudging to work every day and get less and less happy. Sure doesn't sound very appealing. I think it would actually ruin my life.

I have to do something with my life where I feel like I'm making a difference in someone else's life. I know I could do that as a teacher. I can feel now how much it matters to me.

What did I mean by this? How can I describe it more fully?

> I'm a little embarrassed to write this, but I believe I might have a calling to help improve the lives of children. I look at other people who have done this, and I am filled with admiration. These are the people I want to emulate— Fred Rogers, Maria Montessori. I do not want to spend my life making money that only benefits me and my family. I don't mean to say that I have to be some major figure in education; I just feel like I have something unique to offer.

What makes this reason important to me? What would happen if I disregarded it?

> If 50 years from now I have a lot of things, but have not made an impact on a child's life, I think I'll be angry with myself. I'd always wonder what my life could have been like, knowing I may have shortchanged myself as well as the children I could have helped. I also worry that I would feel guilty in the eyes of God if he gave me this calling and I ignored it.

Ellie

My weight casts a shadow over almost everything in my life.

What did I mean by this? How can I describe it more fully?

> I've always been weight conscious, but since I've been heavier it is constantly in the back of my mind, dragging me down.

What makes this reason important to me? What would happen if I disregarded it?

> I am so sick of feeling this way!

I walk into a room, and the first thing I do is check out the size of any female person around my age.

What did I mean by this? How can I describe it more fully?

> I look to see if there's anyone who has thighs as big as mine. If they're thinner than me, I envy them and feel like hiding.

What makes this reason important to me? What would happen if I disregarded it?

> I hate these feelings. They make me feel bad about myself.

I get so self-conscious when there's food around that I try not to eat, and if I do, I'm wondering what people are thinking about me.

What did I mean by this? How can I describe it more fully?

> I think they're thinking, No wonder she looks like that.

What makes this reason important to me? What would happen if I disregarded it?

> It makes me so tense. It's hard to enjoy myself at all. Maybe that's why I spend the whole time in the kitchen and don't let anyone help.

When Gil tries to be affectionate, I don't even want him to touch me.

What did I mean by this? How can I describe it more fully?

> All I can think is, I'm so repulsive—how can he stand to touch me?

What makes this reason important to me? What would happen if I disregarded it?

> I think it makes him feel rejected. He doesn't deserve that.

If I could lose weight, I honestly feel like I'd become almost a different person.

What did I mean by this? How can I describe it more fully?

> I would be happy with myself and comfortable in my own skin. I used to feel more that way when I was younger. It's hard to remember.

What makes this reason important to me? What would happen if I disregarded it?

> I want to see what my life could be like again without these feelings hanging over me.

I could feel more relaxed, even when I'm alone.

What did I mean by this? How can I describe it more fully?

> Part of my brain is in a constant battle over whether I should try to do something about my weight and how to do it if I do try.

What makes this reason important to me? What would happen if I disregarded it?

> It's exhausting. I'm so tired of it.

I could get excited about going clothes shopping for the first time in ages.

What did I mean by this? How can I describe it more fully?

> It used to be fun. I'd even go with my girlfriends. Now it's like a nightmare.

What makes this reason important to me? What would happen if I disregarded it?

> I miss trying something on and liking what I see.

I could look forward to events without stressing over what I'll wear and what I'll look like. I'd be able to socialize with family and friends without feeling so down or uptight.

What did I mean by this? How can I describe it more fully?

> Being this way takes such a toll on me. It sucks a lot of the joy out of my life.

What makes this reason important to me? What would happen if I disregarded it?

> Trying to ignore the problem has made me feel even worse inside.

- -

Often, when people explore the first reasons they thought of for what they believe or how they feel, they find that other reasons begin to emerge as well. So you may already have more "change talk" running through your mind than you've written about. On the other hand, sometimes those other reasons don't come to mind until someone asks us (or we ask ourselves), "*What else* do I think about this?"

So the next step is to read everything you wrote in response to the last activity—the change talk statements you listed and your elaborations on them—out loud and listen to yourself as you're doing it. Then ask yourself, "What else might make me feel that making a change is the right decision for me? What might be some other advantages of change? And what else concerns me when I think about *not* changing? What other disadvantages would there be of leaving things the way they are?"

Consider your companions' responses to these questions, shown below, before you write yours in your journal or the form at *www.guilford. com/zuckoff-forms*.

More Reasons for Change

Alec

What else makes changing right for me? What other advantages might there be?

> Just little things I notice, like not having the energy I used to have in the morning. I don't know how much drinking affects that, but I might feel a little better on days when I haven't had as much the night before. I can't really expect to do what I could do when I was in my 20s. It would be good to feel more alert during the day.

What else concerns me about the status quo? What other disadvantages would there be to keeping it?

> I can't see things getting better between me and Wendy otherwise. Truthfully, some nights I come home later than I have to because I know what I'm going to hear when I get there. I don't want to stay caught in a vicious cycle. It only seems to be getting worse, and I don't like to think about what that could mean.

Barbara

What else makes changing right for me? What other advantages might there be?

> I would no longer be living in this limbo. It feels good now not to be trying to ignore how I feel or what I want, even though it's also scary not knowing what lies ahead. I still don't know what I'm going to do with all this yet, but there's relief in paying attention to it and knowing that I'm going to do something. I feel much more like myself this way, so I must be on the right track.

What else concerns me about the status quo? What other disadvantages would there be to keeping it?

> I think I'd either lose my mind or destroy my marriage. Maybe both. As distracted as he is, I think Steve senses this, too. I know he doesn't want me to be unhappy, but I don't think he can really help me with this situation. I think it is up to me. So as scary as it is to face these decisions instead of talking myself out of them, it's even scarier when I think of doing nothing at all.

Colin

What else makes changing right for me? What other advantages might there be?

> The main thing would be recapturing the way we used to feel and what we were like together before all the fighting started and our relationship began to go bad.

What else concerns me about the status quo? What other disadvantages would there be to keeping it?

> If we broke up I'm not sure I'd ever want to risk getting seriously involved with someone again. I don't know if I could trust this way again. So if I look far into the future, I can see myself alone, and it's not a pretty picture.

Dana

What else makes changing right for me? What other advantages might there be?

> I think it would reconnect me with my friends. I guess I've been avoiding them because they're all so pumped about their careers and I've been feeling crappy about mine—it's hard to be around them. If I was to go for it, I know they'd have my back, unlike my family, so it would be fun to be with them again.

What else concerns me about the status quo? What other disadvantages would there be to keeping it?

> I might start to get bitter or cynical. It's so easy to get caught up in the pettiness and the office gossip where I work. Being unsatisfied plus being in this environment where I don't really fit is a recipe for increased negativity. I worry that I won't like who I become if I stay there.

Ellie

What else makes changing right for me? What other advantages might there be?

> It feels like if I don't try, I'm giving up on myself. Losing weight would give me more energy. I might even try some things for the first time with my husband and kids, like dancing or tennis or some other activity.

What else concerns me about the status quo? What other disadvantages would there be to keeping it?

> I worry that if I don't make some changes, my life will get worse, not stay the same. I could put on even more weight, I could develop health problems, I might even get seriously depressed. That would be really bad for my family, not just me.

Reflecting on the Importance of Change

I'd like to invite you now to reflect on all you've written in response to the activities in this chapter. Please reread your initial response to the question of why you chose the number you did for importance, as well as your further elaborations. If you completed the section exploring the importance of maintaining the status quo, please reread your responses to those questions as well, in the order in which you wrote them (that is, first the explorations of the importance of the status quo and then of the importance of change). How do you feel now about making a change? Use your journal to write your answers or the form "Reflecting on the Importance of Change" at *www.guilford.com/zuckoff-forms*. But first, consider your companions' reflections:

- *Alec:* "When I think about everything in moderation, the idea of making some changes doesn't seem so bad. Somehow this turned into all-or-nothing, and that's where we got stuck. Before I was thinking about how it could get weird if I stopped keeping up when I'm out with customers. But it would be a lot weirder if I had to say 'Nothing for me, I quit.' That's a sobering thought (ha). And if it makes me a little sharper the next day, that would be a bonus. But it's not just the drinking; it's not having any time together that makes Wendy unhappy. So if I could figure out how to have some more down time with her without hurting business, that could start getting us back on a better track. I never wanted my life to be all work and no play."

- *Barbara:* "I kept thinking I had to either push away the feelings I was having or let them push me into something I wasn't ready for. I was terrified I might find out that what I really wanted was something like what Joe was offering and that I would have to leave Steve. Now that I let myself imagine it, I'm sure that sort of excitement is not what I'm looking for. I still don't know what this means for my marriage and my future, but it feels good to know that although I need something to change, it's not that kind of change. So I do feel more like I'm in the driver's seat. But for the first time since my son was born I have no roadmap and the GPS is on the fritz."

- *Colin:* "I feel as though I was attached to a giant rubber band—stretched as far as it could go until it snapped back. I am feeling a little bit better about myself. I hope Paul will be able to understand that I can't take responsibility and work on myself if doing so means that everything bad has been my fault. I think he'll accept that if he sees I understand how much my anger hurts him. And also if I can show him that I'm learning some things about myself, especially about turning him into my enemy when I get angry. So that's my hopeful side. The other side is still there, though. Keeping my integrity but not hurting Paul, and expressing my anger differently—it sounds good, but I don't know if it's possible. I think we'd both have to be working on it, and I don't know how willing he'd be."

- *Dana:* "I want to start seriously researching graduate programs, not just browsing them. Of course, as soon as I write that, this little voice says, 'You're gonna do what?' But now I have an answer—it might be risky, but it's not crazy to consider doing what would make you happy when you're not happy with what you're doing. There are no guarantees in life, except if you get somewhere that's secure and stay there, even if you're miserable! Guaranteed misery—I don't want any part of that. So I'm a little excited but still nervous, especially when I think about how my family might react. I know they want what's best for me, so it's not that they would flip out on me. I don't exactly know what I'm afraid of with them, actually."

- *Ellie:* "It seems to be a no-brainer. I have to face what needs to be done. I don't want to give up on the chance of being satisfied with myself. I definitely don't want things to get worse for me emotionally and physically. And I don't want to keep letting my family down."

REASSESSING IMPORTANCE AFTER LISTENING WITH EARS

My hope is that completing the activities in this chapter has helped you bring your reasons for change (and the feelings associated with them) into sharper relief and weigh their importance to you—and that in doing so your sense of the right direction for you has become clearer. To help you see how much this has happened, I'd like you to rate again the importance to you right now of making a change.

Importance for Chapter 4

How **important** is it to me *right now* to make the change I am considering?

0	1	2	3	4	5	6	7	8	9	10
Not at all					Moderately				Extremely	

First, however, take a look at your companions' ratings and their reasons for choosing the number they did.

Alec, who gave himself a 3 for importance initially and then moved up to a 4, now gives himself a **6:**

> "I could say I was a weak 4, and now I'm a strong 6. The way it looks to me now is that cutting down is the lesser of two evils. I can't say it feels like this big important thing to drink less, but it seems like what I should do. If you were asking me to rate making more time for my wife and daughter to bring down the tension and stress, I'd probably say 7 or 8."

Barbara, who gave herself a 5 for importance initially and then moved up to a 6, now gives herself a **7:**

> "A 7 for knowing with certainty that something is going to change but not knowing yet what that change is going to be."

Colin, who gave himself an 8 for importance initially and then moved down to a 5, now gives himself an **8:**

> "My number at the beginning of this chapter was a fake 5. I didn't want it to be any lower because I'd been trying these different things to get my anger under control and telling myself that I really wanted to do it. I didn't want to admit to myself how ambivalent I was (okay, I'm starting to buy that concept), partly because it was embarrassing, but also because I was scared that if I admitted it, I was really admitting that it was hopeless with Paul, because I was too resentful. Now I'm at a real 8, for me, not for show. I can't lose him."

Dana, who gave herself a 6 for importance initially and then moved up to an 8, now gives herself a **9:**

> "I'm chomping at the bit. I'm separating that from how confident I feel—I can see why you want me to do that, because I still have some doubt about my courage to go all the way through with this, but I have no doubt about what I want and how much it matters to me."

Ellie, who gave herself a 10 for importance initially and then moved down to an 8, now gives herself a **9:**

"A 9 is the closest number to the absolute most important thing in my life, my family. I guess after thinking through all of this, I realize that they are very closely connected. It matters to Gil and even to my kids that I am happy with myself, and it matters to me that I am, too. I feel like I need to do this for all of us."

Now it's time for you to rate yourself again on the same scale. Please circle the number that best captures where you are in terms of the importance of making the change you've been considering, using the rating scale on page 115 and then writing your thoughts about why you chose the number you did in your journal. Or use the form "Importance for Chapter 4" at *www.guilford.com/zuckoff-forms* to circle your importance rating and write down your thoughts about why you chose it.

THE WAY FORWARD

If, like Ellie, you've reached the end of this chapter after already having completed Chapter 5, then please go on to Chapter 6. If, like your other companions, you've not yet completed Chapter 5, it's time to explore more closely "the other half of the battle," your confidence for change. If you find at this point that your importance (or certainty) for changing or staying the same is not yet where it would need to be to get you unstuck, don't be discouraged; in Chapter 6 we will be widening the frame, taking in more of your inner and outer life and helping you place your dilemma in its broader context. For many people, these additional steps are what they need to shift the balance toward resolution of ambivalence.

• • • • 5 • • • •

Exploring Your Confidence for Change

When it comes to resolving ambivalence, half the battle is becoming confident that we can succeed at getting where we want to go. (The other half—finding a way forward whose benefits or advantages dramatically outweigh its costs or disadvantages—is the focus of Chapter 4.) Without that sense of confidence, people have little incentive to commit the energy and effort it takes to change for the better, even when they are sure of the direction they've chosen.

The psychologist Albert Bandura coined the term "self-efficacy"[1] to describe a person's expectation of successfully carrying out an action. His research has shown that we all possess a set of *beliefs* about our abilities and that these beliefs influence our likelihood of success or failure as much as the actual abilities themselves.

For many of the challenges we face, the question that determines our success is not "Can I?" but "Do I believe I can?"

Bandura's research has also shown what creates and shapes those beliefs. The most powerful positive influences on our confidence are

---

[1]Bandura, A. (1997). *Self-efficacy: The exercise of control.* New York: Freeman.

"mastery experiences." These are times when we've faced a situation that we knew would test us and, through effort and persistence, met that challenge successfully. Naturally, the next time we face a similar situation we're more confident that we can handle it. But we don't always transfer that confidence to other situations that, although they may seem different on the surface, could also be met successfully by drawing on the qualities and abilities that helped us master a previous one. Making those connections is one way to increase our confidence in a situation we've not dealt with before.

Another influence on our confidence is how we interpret it when we don't succeed. If we tell ourselves we failed because we lack some inner ability, and there's nothing we can do to replace it, our self-efficacy takes a hit. On the other hand, if we conclude that we fell short because we weren't fully committed, or because we didn't have the tools or resources we needed, we're much more likely to view the outcome as a setback we can overcome with more effort, knowledge, skills, or assistance. Think of a student who gets a bad grade on a test or a chef who gets panned by a critic. The student who thinks, "I'm stupid" or the chef who thinks, "I just don't have what it takes" is going to feel like giving up. But the student who thinks, "I didn't study enough" is likely to redouble his effort the next time around, and the chef who thinks, "I need an expediter in the kitchen so the food goes out perfectly prepared and I can concentrate on cooking" is likely to feel hopeful about taking her restaurant to the next level.

Encouragement and discouragement can also affect our confidence. Interestingly, it is much easier to *decrease* self-efficacy through negative communications than to increase it through positive ones. So as helpful as it can sometimes be to have someone cheering you on, it's even more important to avoid anyone who tends to tell you why you *can't* do something or conveys a message of pessimism about what you're trying to do.

Pep talks pack less of a punch than potshots.

The activities in this chapter are designed to strengthen your belief in your ability to move ahead successfully once you've decided on a direction. To begin, I'd like you to focus on the number you chose on page 89 in answer to the question about your confidence for change and ask yourself why you chose that number rather than a *lower* number. (If you chose 2, why didn't you choose 0? If you chose 5, why not 1 or 2? If you chose 8, why not just 3 or 4?) Then, after you write down the first thing that comes to mind, think about other reasons you chose that number—as many as you can think of.

How your companions responded to these questions is shown below.

. . . .

Why Did I Choose That Number Rather Than a Lower One?

Alec

Confidence = 5

> Cutting back on my drinking doesn't seem too daunting. It won't be easy, but I'm a pretty disciplined guy and I definitely have done harder things in my life. Why else? If making things better at home takes stopping one or two drinks sooner, I guess that's something I can manage. I'm not looking forward to it, though.

Barbara

Confidence = 4

> I feel capable of looking at the situation without such harsh self-judgment. I've been able to remember where my real strengths lie. Now that I feel more resolved that something must change, I feel more in control, even though I still don't know what I need to do. Why else? Because I have always gotten things done in the past and my faith in myself is coming back.

Colin

Confidence = 5

> Making this choice for myself, instead of feeling pressured and resentful, I feel more willing to try. I don't think I'll be able to do it perfectly, but I'll do my part. Remembering how much I don't want to lose him makes me more determined. What else makes me confident? Knowing I want the chance to show him that he was right to fall in love with me in the first place.

Dana

Confidence = 6

> I am a strong and stable person who has done many things responsibly. It's scary, but I am capable of coping with financial challenges. What else? I feel really sure that if I got the chance I could do the job really well. I can't know the future for sure, but I've done pretty well with challenges in my life so far. Why else? Because I am hardworking and a stick-with-it kind of person, and I know I'd give it all I have.

Ellie

Confidence = 2

> Honestly, I'm just trying to hold on to this tiny bit of hope from feeling a little better. But if I actually think about another diet, it seems pointless. I don't want to beat myself up, but how many times can a person go through this?

Now it's your turn. Please ask yourself: "Why did I choose that number, rather than a number that was 2, 3, or 4 *lower?*" That is, "What makes me as confident as I am right now that I could carry out my decision if I knew the choice that is right for me?" Then ask yourself, "Why *else* did I choose that number?" and repeat this process until you cannot think of anything else. (If you chose 0 or 1, and have trouble coming up with reasons to have any confidence at all, don't worry—the special section ahead is just for you.) Enter your answers in your journal or use the form at *www.guilford.com/zuckoff-forms.*

Change Talk or Sustain Talk?

Next I'd like you to mark all the instances of change talk (expressions of self-confidence or belief that you can succeed) and all the instances of sustain talk (expressions of self-doubt or fear that you will fail) in your response. To help you recognize the two types of talk, your companions' responses with change talk highlighted and sustain talk underlined are shown below.

Why Did I Choose That Number Rather Than a Lower One?

Alec

Confidence = 5

> Cutting back on my drinking doesn't seem too daunting. It won't be easy, but I'm a pretty disciplined guy, and I definitely have done harder things in my life. Why else? If making things better at home takes stopping one or two drinks sooner, I guess that's something I can manage. I'm not looking forward to it, though.

Barbara

Confidence = 4

I feel capable of looking at the situation without such harsh self-judgment. I've been able to remember where my real strengths lie. Now that I feel more resolved that something must change, I feel more in control, even though I still don't know what I need to do. Why else? Because I have always gotten things done in the past and my faith in myself is coming back.

Colin

Confidence = 5

Making this choice for myself, instead of feeling pressured and resentful, I feel more willing to try. I don't think I'll be able to do it perfectly, but I'll do my part. Remembering how much I don't want to lose him makes me more determined. What else makes me confident? Knowing I want the chance to show him that he was right to fall in love with me in the first place.

Dana

Confidence = 6

I am a strong and stable person who has done many things responsibly. It's scary, but I am capable of coping with financial challenges. What else? I feel really sure that if I got the chance, I could do the job really well. I can't know the future for sure, but I've done pretty well with challenges in my life so far. Why else? Because I am hardworking and a stick-with-it kind of person, and I know I'd give it all I have.

Ellie

Confidence = 2

Honestly, I'm just trying to hold on to this tiny bit of hope from feeling a little better. But if I actually think about another diet, it seems pointless. I don't want to beat myself up, but how many times can a person go through this?

- -

Now it's your turn. Please mark all the instances of change talk and all the instances of sustain talk in your response. If you're not sure whether something you wrote is change talk or sustain talk, leave it unmarked; if you think it might be both, mark it as both. If you're highlighting, use different colors so you can easily identify the two kinds of talk. If you're using pencil or pen, circle the change talk and underline the sustain talk.

Just like your companions, it's likely that your response included both change talk and sustain talk. This is not at all surprising; not yet having met the challenge, it makes sense that you would have some uncertainty about success. If you found at least some change talk in your response, please skip the next section and go on to "Exploring Your Confidence for Change." However, if, like Ellie's, your response was pessimistic or focused on failure, then please continue on to the next section.

YOUR PESSIMISM ABOUT CHANGE

When I invited you to think about the strengths and resources you can draw on when you know what you want to accomplish, you found yourself thinking about your inability to change.

One reason that can happen is actually related more to importance than to confidence. When a person has significant doubts about pursuing a course of action, those doubts can "bleed over" and affect confidence as well. After all, one thing that bolsters our confidence is knowing that the benefits of change so far outweigh the costs that we are willing to persevere no matter how difficult things get and make accomplishing it a high priority.

Some years ago Sara, a woman in a therapy group with me, told the group that she had wanted to end her marriage for several years. Her husband had become increasingly preoccupied with his hobbies and emotionally distant; their sex life had ended years before. She'd tried everything she could to find out from him what had changed without success, and he'd adamantly refused couple counseling. She wondered whether he was having an affair but saw no sign of it and thought it more likely that he had just lost interest in her. Despite her intention to leave, though, she had never been able to find the courage and the means to do it.

Members of the group offered encouragement as well as practical support, which she accepted with appreciation but without any discernible effect on her confidence. Although she had expressed certainty about what she wanted and asked for help, when I asked her to say more about her reasons for wanting to leave, she initially talked about her unhappiness in the marriage but then began to talk about what her husband meant to her. She had grown up in a neglectful and emotionally barren family, she told us, and had left home when she was young to be with him, the only person she'd ever felt cared for her. She felt he had rescued her, and in the next few years she had learned to trust another person for the first time. When she thought back to that time, she continued to feel a deep sense of gratitude toward him.

As Sara described her memories of their marriage in its first years, I wondered aloud how she would feel about herself if she did, finally, leave him. "Like an ungrateful child," she said, and then after a pause, "I guess I've been feeling that way ever since I started thinking about separating." When I asked her to imagine that, somehow, she no longer felt that way, she immediately responded, "Then nothing would stop me." It was clear to all, including Sara, that her apparently low confidence in her ability to leave and make it on her own had everything to do with these unspoken reservations about her decision.

So imagine, hypothetically, that you knew with 100% certainty—no doubts at all—the right decision for you and what you want to accomplish. How confident (on the 0–10 scale) would you be that you could make that change right now? If the number you choose is significantly higher than the one you chose at the end of the First Interlude, please go back to Chapter 4. After you have completed the activities there designed to help you explore the importance of the change you're considering, come back to this chapter, starting with the next section, "Exploring Your Confidence for Change." (If your confidence level rose significantly, but you *have* already completed Chapter 4, please continue with this section; in Chapter 6 you will find more help in coming to a firm decision about what your way forward should be.)

If, like Ellie, your number for confidence stayed the same, it's very likely that repeated, unsuccessful efforts to change your behavior or situation over an extended period have left you feeling discouraged. It might be that this is not the only change you have found it frustratingly difficult to make. Perhaps you've been led to believe, from messages you've received from others (including some of the important people in your life), that you don't have what it takes to make things better for yourself.

Whatever the source of the hopelessness you are feeling, I believe change is possible for you, no matter who you are or how you see yourself. My confidence comes from the many people I have worked with individually, who came to me similarly despairing about their ability to improve their situation and yet were ultimately able to find what they needed within themselves to make change happen.

One client in particular stands out in memory: Donal, a middle-aged man who came for help with his drug use. In our first meeting, he told me that he had begun drinking when he was a teenager and then added regular use of marijuana, cocaine, and opiate medications in quick succession as he tried to comfort himself during an adolescence filled with loneliness and neglect. He related how, over the previous 2 years, he had weaned himself off everything except for marijuana—which he now smoked all the time. Not only did he feel helpless to stop, despite repeated efforts to do so, but unlike the other substances he had used, he could not imagine his life without marijuana.

A few months after that first meeting, Donal achieved abstinence from marijuana without returning to the use of any other drugs. I'll return to Donal's story in Part III, when we focus on developing workable and effective plans for change. But I mention him now to lend you my hope, by pointing out what you and he have in common. Despite your strong and convincing doubts about your ability to solve your dilemma, you have not given up—you have continued to seek someone or something to help you overcome the obstacles you face. And the question I'd like you to ask yourself now is: "Why *haven't* I given up? What has given me the strength to keep on trying in the face of what might seem like overwhelming odds?" But first consider Ellie's answers to these questions, shown below.

. . . .

Why Haven't I Given Up?

Ellie

> Because I don't want to feel like a failure. I don't want to accept that I have to live like this until I die. I believe deep inside that I should be able to be happy with who I am, and even though I feel funny saying it, that I deserve to feel that way. And maybe because I know I'm stronger than I sometimes give myself credit for.

. . . .

Now it's your turn. Enter your response in your journal or use the form at *www.guilford.com/zuckoff-forms*. If, like Ellie, your response includes positive thoughts about your ability to change, please highlight the change talk as shown for Ellie below.

. . . .

Why Haven't I Given Up?

Ellie

> Because I don't want to feel like a failure. I won't accept that I have to live like this until I die. I believe deep inside that I should be able to be happy with who I am, and even though I feel funny saying it, that I deserve to feel that way. And maybe because I know I'm stronger than I sometimes give myself credit for.

. . . .

EXPLORING YOUR CONFIDENCE FOR CHANGE

Please list each instance of change talk in your response at the beginning of this chapter and in your response to the question of why you haven't given up, if you completed it. How you group or separate them is up to you; there's no right or wrong way. It's fine to break up sentences if different parts of a sentence mean different things to you. If you want to do it the way your companions did, shown below, you can use the form at *www. guilford.com/zuckoff-forms*, or write in your journal any way you like. Then ask yourself these questions about each one:

- "What did I mean by this? How can I describe it more fully?"
- "What does this say about my ability to accomplish a difficult change?"

- -

My Ability to Change

Alec

Cutting back on my drinking doesn't seem too daunting. I have definitely done harder things in my life.

What did I mean by this? How can I describe it more fully?

> I was on the track team in college, and those guys were drinkers. But when we were training and we had to cut back, we did it. It was more of a struggle getting my weight down because of the junk food we lived on, but I did that, too. I wasn't going to let myself or the team down.

What does this say about my ability to accomplish a difficult change?

> That if I want something badly enough I will sacrifice for it.

I'm a pretty disciplined guy.

What did I mean by this? How can I describe it more fully?

> I could not have achieved what I have in life if I wasn't able to focus and get things done.

What does this say about my ability to accomplish a difficult change?

> If I decide to do this, I can make it happen.

If making things better at home takes stopping one or two drinks sooner, I guess that's something I can manage.

What did I mean by this? How can I describe it more fully?

> Maybe I've been making more out of this than I needed to. Maybe it's been more about not knuckling under than how it will affect work.

What does this say about my ability to accomplish a difficult change?

> When I put it that way, it doesn't sound like such a big deal. I don't know if that'll be enough for Wendy, though.

Barbara

I feel capable of looking at the situation without such harsh self-judgment.

What did I mean by this? How can I describe it more fully?

> Being so hard on myself made it impossible to think straight. So I was robbing myself of one of my greatest assets.

What does this say about my ability to accomplish a difficult change?

> Now that I can sort through all these different feelings I should be able to make sense of them.

I've been able to remember where my real strengths lie. My faith in myself is coming back. I have always gotten things done in the past.

What did I mean by this? How can I describe it more fully?

> I am very good at looking at a situation, analyzing what is needed, coming up with a plan, and carrying it out. Remembering that makes me feel less overwhelmed even though I don't have an answer yet.

What does this say about my ability to accomplish a difficult change?

> It tells me that I don't have to be so afraid. If I rely on my strengths, I can handle this.

Now that I feel more resolved that something must change, I feel more in control.

What did I mean by this? How can I describe it more fully?

> I felt out of control because the feelings I was having wouldn't go away, no matter how much I tried to talk myself out of them.

What does this say about my ability to accomplish a difficult change?

> Trying to convince myself that I can accept things I can't accept won't solve anything. Tackling them head-on will, I hope.

Colin

Making this choice for myself, instead of feeling pressured and resentful, I'm more willing to try.

What did I mean by this? How can I describe it more fully?

> I can see now why I've had such a hard time restraining my anger: my heart wasn't completely in it.

What does this say about my ability to accomplish a difficult change?

> I'm only going to be able to do this if I do it wholeheartedly. If I'm really willing, I should be able to find a way.

I will do my part.

What did I mean by this? How can I describe it more fully?

> It matters to me to be the kind of person who will meet someone at least halfway. "Take me or leave me" won't work, but neither will "You're all wrong and I'm all right." There are things we both need to work on.

What does this say about my ability to accomplish a difficult change?

> As long as I'm not alone in this, and I'm not expected to be perfect, I think I can figure out how to do it.

Remembering how much I don't want to lose him makes me more determined.

What did I mean by this? How can I describe it more fully?

> I was so focused on what I was supposed to be doing with my anger that I stopped thinking about why it mattered.

What does this say about my ability to accomplish a difficult change?

> Keeping how important Paul is to me at the forefront of my mind should give me the motivation I need to do what's hard for me.

I want the chance to show him that he was right to fall in love with me in the first place.

What did I mean by this? How can I describe it more fully?

> *I don't like that Paul sees me as less than how he saw me when we were first together. I want him to see me as special again.*

What does this say about my ability to accomplish a difficult change?

> *Pride gets a bad rap, but it can motivate you. It's not a big part of it, but I guess it's there.*

Dana

I am a strong and stable person. I've done pretty well with challenges in my life so far.

What did I mean by this? How can I describe it more fully?

> *I was thinking about some of the things I've had to cope with in my life. Being able to handle a lot of stress is my gift, and it has helped me through tough times.*

What does this say about my ability to accomplish a difficult change?

> *No matter how much upheaval there might be if I do this, I know I'll be able to handle it.*

. . . who has done many things responsibly.

What did I mean by this? How can I describe it more fully?

> *I'm the opposite of impulsive. I look before I leap, consider the consequences, and think about others' needs before I do anything.*

What does this say about my ability to accomplish a difficult change?

> *If I decide to do this, it will be a responsible decision. Knowing that makes me feel a little less scared.*

I am capable of coping with financial challenges.

What did I mean by this? How can I describe it more fully?

> *I know how to live without luxuries and get by on what I have.*

What does this say about my ability to accomplish a difficult change?

> *I will need this skill if I become a student again. I will be able to manage it.*

. . . if I got the chance, I could do the job really well.

What did I mean by this? How can I describe it more fully?

> This is what I was saying before—I know I have what it takes to be a good teacher, the ability and the passion.

What does this say about my ability to accomplish a difficult change?

> Loving what you do increases the chances that you'll succeed.

I am hardworking and a stick-with-it kind of person. I know I'd give it all I have.

What did I mean by this? How can I describe it more fully?

> When things get hard, I work harder. I've never given up on anything I wanted, even when I was scared. Why should this be any different?

What does this say about my ability to accomplish a difficult change?

> When I think about how well I've done at a job I never loved, I think, "What will you be able to do when you are doing something you love?"

Ellie

I won't accept that I have to live like this until I die.

What did I mean by this? How can I describe it more fully?

> It makes me mad to think of myself spending my whole adult life worrying about my weight. What a waste!

What does this say about my ability to accomplish a difficult change?

> I'll never really resign myself to being fat. So either I find some way to do something about it or I will keep making myself miserable.

I believe deep inside that I should be able to be happy with who I am. I deserve to feel that way.

What did I mean by this? How can I describe it more fully?

> This is what I don't usually let myself think about. Maybe because I don't want to be mad at anybody for not helping me more. Which would be totally unfair, because I don't let anybody help me even if they want to.

What does this say about my ability to accomplish a difficult change?

> I might have to let people help me. That feels uncomfortable, even though I'm always telling the clients I work with that there's nothing shameful about asking for help because everybody needs help sometimes.

I know I'm stronger than I sometimes give myself credit for.

What did I mean by this? How can I describe it more fully?

> Taking care of my family and giving to others shows strength, especially when they're hurting and they need support. So is working as hard as I do and not complaining about it.

What does this say about my ability to accomplish a difficult change?

> I need to stop forgetting this. If I'm going to have any chance of losing weight for good, I'm going to need all the strength I can find.

Building Confidence from Past Success

I noted at the beginning of this chapter that it's common to miss out on a powerful source of confidence for addressing a dilemma: successes you've had in dealing with other kinds of challenges in the past. Because those situations may seem quite different from the one you're working on, it may not have occurred to you that the same qualities and strengths that made the difference then can also help you now, once you are aware enough to tap into them.

So I'd like you to describe a situation in the past in which you overcame a difficult challenge and ask yourself the following questions about it:

- "Which of my strengths or qualities made it possible for me to succeed? What were the most important contributors to my success?"
- "How could those strengths or qualities apply to the dilemma I am facing now? How could I use them to change my current situation if I decided change was the right decision for me?"

Before writing your answers in your journal or in the form at *www.guilford.com/zuckoff-forms* consider your companions' answers, shown below.

A Difficult Challenge I Overcame

Alec

The challenge I overcame was:

> Talking about my days of running track: I was running trails with my buddies and heard a snap followed by excruciating pain. I had torn my hamstring, and the way I fell messed my leg up. It was a full tear that needed surgery and a six-month recovery and physical therapy.

What contributed most to my success? What strengths or qualities made it possible?

> More than anything, I guess you'd call it determination. Or maybe mule-headedness. When I asked the surgeon if I'd be as good as I was before the surgery, he said, "It's possible," like he didn't mean it. I swore to myself, "It's not possible, it's happening." I worked like crazy, every day. I had to tolerate a lot of pain. But the hardest part was probably not pushing ahead too fast and reinjuring myself. Patience was never my strong suit, but I had to learn some.

How could those strengths or qualities apply to the dilemma I am facing now? How could I use them in my current situation?

> I don't think I ever wanted anything so much in my life as I wanted to run again. And I did it. So I'm starting to see how that applies here. How much do I want my good life with my wife back? If I want it enough, I'll be disciplined enough to cut back and tolerate some uncomfortable feelings. Plus, it wouldn't happen overnight, so I'd have to use my patience while we tried to get back on a better track.

Barbara

The challenge I overcame was:

> A few years ago my mother-in-law came to stay with us while she was recovering from a fall. She can be lovely, but her tendency to be critical and demanding was magnified tenfold and I was first in the line of fire. I did not want to do anything that would have a negative impact on our relationship, and that was quite the challenge. Two of the kids were still at home, and Steve was working long hours. She was with us for 3 weeks, but it seemed much longer.

What contributed most to my success? What strengths or qualities made it possible?

> I reminded myself that I was doing this by choice. I offered because I liked her and wanted to be a good daughter-in-law. When I kept that in mind, it was easier to let her remarks roll off me. And I kept my sense of humor. I remember my daughter saying she thought it was cool that I could get Grandma to laugh when she was so crabby! Steve was the only one who knew how challenging it was, and he really appreciated me for being so generous with her.

How could those strengths or qualities apply to the dilemma I am facing now? How could I use them in my current situation?

> Focusing on having a choice might help. Feeling pushed around by all my emotions and worries was scary. The feelings aren't of my choosing, but what I do about them can be—that makes me feel saner. And I might be able

to take a step back and find some humor in this whole fiasco. Nothing lowers my stress level better than when I can find some absurdity in a situation and even poke fun at myself. Maybe I need a night out with my sister just to laugh with each other!

Colin

The challenge I overcame was:

When I was in art school, I had the opportunity to study abroad in Paris. Unfortunately, I had no money and I could not speak French. So I had one summer to earn enough cash and learn to speak a foreign language well enough to get by. I used every spare minute and every ounce of my creativity to make it possible. I worked two jobs and spent all my free time studying French. And I went to France and it was one of the best experiences of my life.

What contributed most to my success? What strengths or qualities made it possible?

Determination, of course, but also creativity. There's no way I would've learned what I did from a textbook. I taped notes on every item in my house, I listened to recordings of songs that I knew, but in French, I recorded my own songs in French, I watched French films with subtitles . . . you could call it ingenuity, too.

How could those strengths or qualities apply to the dilemma I am facing now? How could I use them in my current situation?

Determination I already knew about, but I hadn't thought about creativity in this situation. All along I've been doing the standard anger-management things. It never occurred to me that I could be creative in coming up with fresh ways to handle my feelings with Paul. I like that.

Dana

The challenge I overcame was:

Physics in my senior year of high school was very hard for me. I knew I wanted a higher grade than a C in the class, but I was just not getting it, and I didn't know what to do.

What contributed most to my success? What strengths or qualities made it possible?

I was shy, but I got up the courage to meet with the teacher after class. At first I was so intimidated by him I didn't want to ask questions for fear of looking dumb, but I kept meeting with him, and I got a tutor as well. I studied hard, and when I got a B− on the midterm, I asked the teacher if I could do extra credit. He let everyone do that, and I saw that others were

> struggling, too. I joined a study group, did extra credit work, and ended up getting an A– in the class!

How could those strengths or qualities apply to the dilemma I am facing now? How could I use them in my current situation?

> I will need to rely on my courage if I decide to go back to school, even when talking with my family. I am better at seeking help now than I was at that age; I've learned it's often necessary, not just for me. I've been thinking about looking into financial aid and finding out about how graduate students manage. Being willing to put in extra work is definitely a quality I would need to use, maybe even getting a part-time job if it's allowed.

Ellie

The challenge I overcame was:

> When my sister was getting married, I panicked at having to fly to be there. I had never been in an airplane. I wanted to rent a car and drive! Neither of us had jobs where we could take time off to drive there and back. I couldn't miss my sister's wedding, so I knew I had to do it.

What contributed most to my success? What strengths or qualities made it possible?

> The main thing that helped me do this was Gil's support and encouragement. He told me to read up on how airplanes work and how risky flying actually is. He spent a lot of time listening to my fears and literally and figuratively held my hand through the entire ordeal. My love for my sister was also crucial. I knew how hurt and disappointed she'd be if I wasn't there, and I refused to do that to her. I would have regretted it forever if I'd missed it. Even so, I still had to screw up my courage to get on that plane.

How could those strengths or qualities apply to the dilemma I am facing now? How could I use them in my current situation?

> Trusting Gil enough to provide help when I need it used to be more of a strength. I think I've shut him out when it comes to my weight. Maybe I need to rethink that. My willingness to fight through feeling uncomfortable for the sake of the people I love is also a strength. Then again, even though I never give in to the temptation to skip an event because I cannot find anything to wear that does not look like a tent, I do have a hard time relaxing once I'm there. So reminding myself that feeling better about my weight would make me more fun to be around might give me more motivation. For sure, it would take all my courage to try this one more time.

REASSESSING CONFIDENCE AFTER LISTENING WITH EARS

Please read out loud everything you wrote in response to the last two activities: the change talk statements you listed from the beginning of this chapter and your elaborations on them as well as your recollections of the difficult challenge you overcame.

Have the activities in this chapter helped to strengthen your belief in your own ability to change? If you were certain about the change you wanted to make, how confident are you right now that you would be able to do it?

. . . .

Confidence for Chapter 5

How **confident** am I *right now* that I would be able to make that change?

0	1	2	3	4	5	6	7	8	9	10
Not at all					Moderately				Extremely	

. . . .

Here are your companions' ratings and their reasons for choosing the number they did.

Alec, who gave himself a 9 for confidence initially and then moved down to a 4, now gives himself a 7:

> "It's hard to say you know you can do something when you're not sure you want to do it, right? When I start to think about the nuts and bolts of what it would take to cut down my drinking, it's pretty clear that it's doable if I decide to make it happen. But I'm still going to have to see how slowing down and coming home earlier is going to work and if it's enough to get Wendy and me back on the same side."

Barbara, who gave herself a 2 for confidence initially and then moved up to a 4, now gives herself a 6:

> "The more I get in touch with my own strengths and personality, the more hopeful I feel. I need to not only lighten up on myself but also add some levity back into my life. I'm going to find my way through this, and I don't have to panic."

Colin, who gave himself a 7 for confidence initially and then moved down to a 5, now gives himself a **7**:

> "I've been looking at the situation through the same lens for such a long time, and suddenly it looks different. I'm almost excited about coming up with creative solutions."

Dana, who gave herself a 4 for confidence initially and then moved up to a 6, now gives herself an **8**:

> "I don't have to keep doubting my own judgment, because I know I make good decisions. I'm not feeling worried and afraid anymore; more nervous about stepping out of my secure world to do what I feel called to do and explaining it to my parents."

Ellie, who gave herself a 0 for confidence initially and then moved up to a 2, now gives herself a **4**:

> "I'm starting to think I've been trying to lose weight with one hand tied behind my back (and not to stop me from eating, ha!). I wasn't always unwilling to let Gil help me. I forgot how supportive he can be and how important that was. I have not been giving him the credit he deserves. Or myself, for that matter. When it comes to something that matters this much to me and actually hurts the quality of the time I spend with my family, I need to ask for help."

Now it's time for you to rate yourself again on the same scale. Please circle the number that best captures where you are in terms of your confidence for making the change you've been considering, using the rating scale on page 135 or the form "Confidence for Chapter 5" at *www.guilford. com/zuckoff-forms*. Then write down your thoughts about why you chose the number you did, using your journal or the online form.

THE WAY FORWARD

If, like Ellie, you're completing this chapter before Chapter 4, you will shortly be returning there to explore the importance of change for you. If you've already completed Chapter 4, you will next move to Chapter 6, where we will focus on the role of attention to your personal values in helping you get unstuck. However, first I'd like you to complete one more activity related to your confidence for change, to plant a seed that we will seek to nurture further if and when you become ready to start planning for whatever change you've decided to make.

Thinking about your level of confidence for change right now, ask yourself what you would need to feel *more* confident. (If you're at a 2, what would help you move up to 4 or 5? If you're at a 4, what would help you move up to 6 or 7? If you're at a 7, what would help you reach 8 or 9?) What would make a difference in how able you feel to pursue your chosen path?

Consider your companions' responses, which appear below, before entering your own in your journal or the form at *www.guilford.com/zuckoff-forms*.

. . . .

What Would I Need to Feel More Confident?

Alec

Confidence = 7

> I don't know yet if the changes I'm thinking about making would be enough to make things better between Wendy and me. If they worked, they would feel more important, and that would make me more determined to keep it up. I guess if I tried it out to see if it makes a difference with her, or even with my energy level in the mornings, I could see what happened. But maybe I'd want to talk to her and see if she is on board first, to see if it's worth it to put the work in.

Barbara

Confidence = 6

> I would have to have a clearer sense of direction. I'm feeling more hopeful, but I still don't know what I can do to put that challenge and excitement back into my life without leaving Steve. Maybe I need to spend some time with myself now that I'm feeling more like myself. Or maybe talk with my sister about what I'm thinking and see if she can help.

Colin

Confidence = 7

> I'm nervous about how Paul will react when I talk to him about what I've been thinking. He's been pretty clear that it's my responsibility to get my anger under control and I don't know how he'll feel about me trying to

> explain why I need him to help me feel like I'm not the bad guy and tell me what kinds of expressions of anger are okay for me to do. If he understands and wants to support me in changing, I will be much more confident about doing it.

Dana

Confidence = 8

> To be totally confident I'd probably have to start gathering detailed information about different programs, application requirements and deadlines, costs, and so on. I'd have to start narrowing down my options and finding out what steps I'd have to take. And I'd need to think about exactly how I would break the news to my parents, what I would say to them and where and when I would say it. Wow. I'm starting to sound really serious!

Ellie

Confidence = 4

> I have a long way to go before I could actually feel confident about losing weight. I'd have to have a weight loss plan I believe in, and I'm nowhere near that now. But you didn't ask me what would make me a 10, right? So, to be a little more confident, I guess I'd have to talk to Gil. Maybe test the waters to see his reactions. I'm not sure I'm ready for that, though.

What You Need and How to Get It

Like your companions, many people find that it's only once they've begun to work on changing and start to see progress that their confidence in their ultimate success reaches its peak. Naturally, developing a plan for change that you believe will work and the readiness to put it into action must come first, like the horse before the cart. And part of developing such a plan is thinking more about how to find the help you need. All of which is by way of saying that once you are ready to move ahead, we'll use your understanding of what you'll need to carry out change as the jumping-off point for helping you get it. But for now, there is one last step to strengthen your conviction about the path ahead of you.

• • • • 6 • • • •

Exploring Your Personal Values

My coauthor, Bonnie, smoked her first cigarette in college. It started as something to do at parties or when hanging out with friends. In time, however, what began as a minor enhancement to her social activities became a stress reliever she relied on. Though she never became a "heavy" smoker, when life felt challenging, cigarettes were a source of relaxation. When things were calmer, she would quit, for up to a year at a time, for all the obvious reasons: the health risks, the cost of a pack, even the smell on her clothes. Yet she would always resume regular smoking when that "special friend" was needed.

As her 20s gave way to her 30s, cigarettes became increasingly woven into the fabric of Bonnie's life, and more and more time went by without the familiar "Time to quit!" feeling arising. Instead, a vague sense crept up on her that smoking was taking hold of her in a way that it hadn't before. She pushed that awareness away, telling herself that she would know when the time was right. She also tried not to notice that she was smoking more than she ever had.

One motive these days for quitting smoking that was *not* a factor at that time (the late 1980s) is the diminishing availability of places where one can smoke undisturbed. Back then, Bonnie could light up without a thought at the college counseling center where she worked; at meetings, she and the center's director would lay out their respective packs and ashtrays, alternately holding their pens to take notes and dragging on their burning cigarettes.

During her first few months at the counseling center Bonnie had come to rely heavily on the center's administrative assistant, Kylie, a smart, efficient, assertive, socially savvy woman with a strong moral code that she followed unwaveringly. Able to anticipate the needs of those around her with startling accuracy, Kylie was indispensable to the center. She had also become Bonnie's close and deeply respected friend.

One afternoon, Kylie entered Bonnie's office and closed the door behind her. With tears in her eyes, she said her mother had been diagnosed with cancer and there was little hope for her survival. She talked with a mixture of frustration and anguish about her mother's love of cigarettes and how she had resisted Kylie's pleadings to give them up.

In the days that followed, Bonnie watched as Kylie came to work and did her job as she always had, though with an aura of sadness that grew with each passing week. From time to time Kylie would enter Bonnie's office, close the door, and talk about her mother's treatment and the prospect of losing her. For Bonnie it would have been impossible to light a cigarette during these talks, out of sensitivity to Kylie's struggle. But from her empathy for Kylie and her family's situation Bonnie felt something inside begin to change. An appreciation for the simple fact of her own physical well-being, of being humbled by her good fortune, began to grow, and along with it the feeling that it was wrong for her to be smoking at all—as though it were an insult to anyone who did not have the good health she enjoyed to treat it so cavalierly. She felt a deepening awareness of the value of her own life, even of life itself, which finally resulted in the realization that not only did she want to quit, but that she had to.

When she told Kylie about her decision, and that it had been inspired by her respect for Kylie and her mom, Bonnie could see how touched Kylie was. She stopped smoking soon after. It was harder than it had been in the past; the nicotine cravings were intense, and in almost every situation she had the thought that a cigarette would make it better. But she knew deep inside that this time she was quitting for good. More than 25 years later, Bonnie remains an ex-smoker.

VALUES: THE ENGINE OF CHANGE

Values are our beliefs about how we should live and our aspirations for who we want to be. Our values shape our attitudes and opinions about others' behavior as well as our own; they are the principles that guide us when we're trying to decide whether an action is right or wrong or whether a situation we encounter is desirable or undesirable.

Many of the values people hold come from the family, culture, and religious tradition in which they were raised. Some accept and preserve those values largely as they were passed down. Others may intentionally explore, rework, and in some cases replace those values with ones of their own choosing. Many people find that their values change gradually, as life experiences lead them to new judgments about what really matters.

Unlike our goals, which we may be able to reach through our efforts and which, once met, no longer play a direct role in our choices, we never finally "achieve" our values. If I have a goal of getting a particular job, then once I've been hired that goal will give way to a new goal—perhaps doing well enough to earn a promotion or to carve out a niche as a valued employee. But there's no point when we can say, "Okay, now I'm honest— that's done." Living out, and living up to, our personal values is a lifelong process that we can never perfect, especially as our values shift and we find ourselves acting on new principles and priorities that emerge along the way.

Values Can Guide Our Decisions about Change

Bonnie's story illustrates several reasons why a focus on personal values is a central component of the process of resolving ambivalence. When people's *core values*—their most fundamental, deeply held beliefs about what it means to be a good person and live a good life—are brought to the fore, a sudden shift in how they view the situation they are in and their place in it may occur, which in turn can trigger resolution of even long-standing ambivalence about change. A sense of reverence for life and gratitude for what it had given her were part of who Bonnie was. Yet it was not until she came face to face with her friend's pain at losing what was most precious to her and saw herself implicated in the source of that pain, through her continued use of tobacco, that the balance between the "good" things and the "not-so-good things" about smoking was definitively tipped.

Bonnie's sudden shift also highlights the fact that values are not the only influences on the choices we make. Smoking was not consistent with Bonnie's core values—but continuing to smoke was the path of least resistance for her, and in the absence of anything to bring those values to the front of her mind, its everyday benefits were substantial enough to keep her lighting up, despite the vague discomfort that accompanied the behavior.

The effects of listening to ourselves on how we understand ourselves are also apparent in Bonnie's story. We may not know exactly what our values are, or what they mean to us, until we put them into

Our deepest values can guide us in our hardest decisions . . . but only if we're conscious of them.

words. Or, to paraphrase: in part, we learn what we value as we hear ourselves speak. Through her conversations with Kylie, Bonnie discovered what mattered most to her.

Conflicting Values Can Keep Us Stuck

There is one more point I want to make about how values shape our attitudes and actions, which was brought home by a client named John during a values exploration activity quite similar to the one I will be guiding you through in this chapter.

Like Bonnie, John was a smoker, and he expressed a longtime, unfulfilled desire to quit. When asked to say more about why he wanted to stop smoking, John emphasized that, as a respiratory therapist, he felt hypocritical engaging in a behavior that he frequently sought to help his patients eliminate. As he was otherwise quite focused on maintaining a healthy lifestyle, conscious of acting in ways consistent with his values, and disciplined in his behavior, he was more than a little mystified (and embarrassed) about his continuing inability to give up cigarettes despite multiple attempts to do so.

John identified health ("to be physically well and healthy"), excitement ("to have a life full of thrills and stimulation"), and authenticity ("to be true to who I am") as his core values. When asked what each of these values meant to him, John began by talking about the high priority he placed on taking care of himself physically. This went beyond a basic concern for his health; John took seriously the biblical mandate to view his body as a temple, and he believed that treating it with respect was a way not only to increase his chances for a long and vital life, but also to honor his creator.

The incongruity of smoking for John was apparent, until he turned his attention to the value he placed on excitement. When he was younger, he said, taking care of his health also allowed him to push his body to its limits through participation in extreme sports, which made him feel alive and on the edge. As he grew older and more settled, he found fewer and fewer opportunities to have those kinds of experiences.

As John spoke about the way his life had changed, the thought struck him that smoking was perhaps the only way, in his otherwise well-ordered and responsible existence, he could still regularly experience a sense of doing something risky, even putting his life on the line. John sat in silence for several moments after sharing this realization, and then, in a quiet voice, went on, "No wonder I haven't been able to quit."

The outcome of John's values exploration illustrates how a person can remain stuck in ambivalence because, without being aware of it, the very behavior his values tell him to change is also one that his values tell him to continue. One of the most difficult aspects of being human is that we possess multiple values, some of which may conflict. In many cases we hold these values in hierarchies, or orders of importance—so that, for example, if I value winning, but I value honesty more, I can resist the temptation to cheat at cards without regretting the lost hands it might cost me. But some of us, like John, perceive a conflict between two of our core values, neither of which can be ignored without creating a feeling of violating our own principles—and in John's case, his own core value of authenticity as well.

When our deepest values are in conflict, our actions leave us unsatisfied with ourselves until we bring them into harmony.

Psychologist Milton Rokeach, who studied the relationship between values and behavior,[1] called the feeling generated by such conflicts, and the recognition that we are not living out our values as fully as we would wish, "self-dissatisfaction" and pointed out that it troubles us as much as it does because it represents a threat to our positive overall view of ourselves—the need for self-esteem that, along with the desire to feel in control of our own actions, lies at the heart of human motivation. Through this chapter's activities, I will help you bring your core values to bear on the dilemma you have been struggling with by listening to yourself as you identify them, describe their unique meanings for you, and consider their implications for the choice you are facing. I will also help you recognize whether your struggle is being made harder by a conflict among your core values, and if so, to begin to think about how to honor both of those values instead of having to choose between them.

IDENTIFYING AND EXPLORING YOUR VALUES

What Are the Values That Matter to You?

On pages 144–146 you will find a list of values, each one briefly defined, adapted from a list developed by Bill Miller and colleagues.[2] Read through the list and circle each word that names a value that is important to you; you can use the form at *www.guilford.com/zuckoff-forms* if you like. Choose only those that genuinely matter to you and not what you or others think

---

[1]Rokeach, M. (1973). *The nature of human values.* New York: Free Press.

[2]Miller, W. R., C'de Baca, J., Matthews, D. B., & Wilbourne, P. L. (2001). *Personal values card sort.* Albuquerque: University of New Mexico. Available at *http://casaa.unm. edu/inst/Personal%20Values%20Card%20Sort.pdf.*

you *should* value (but don't). There's no "right" or "wrong" number, so don't worry if you're circling too many or too few. I've left some blanks at the bottom for you to add any values you hold that I haven't listed.

My Personal Values

Acceptance to be accepted as I am	**Achievement** to have important accomplishments
Admiration to be looked up to and held in high regard	**Adventure** to have new and exciting experiences
Attractiveness to be physically attractive	**Authenticity** to be true to who I am
Authority to be in charge of and responsible for others	**Autonomy** to determine my own actions
Beauty to appreciate beauty around me	**Belonging** to feel like a part of something
Caring to take care of others	**Challenge** to take on difficult tasks and problems
Comfort to have a pleasant and comfortable life	**Commitment** to devote myself to something and stick with it
Compassion to feel and act on concern for others	**Confidence** to feel sure of myself and know I can succeed
Contribution to add something to the world	**Cooperation** to work well together with others
Creativity to have original ideas and create new things	**Dependability** to be reliable and trustworthy
Duty to carry out my duties and obligations	**Ecology** to take care of the environment

Excitement to have a life full of thrills and stimulation	**Fame** to be known and recognized
Family to have a happy, loving family X	**Fitness** to be physically fit and strong
Forgiveness to forgive and be forgiven X	**Friendship** X to have close, supportive friends
Fun X to play and have fun	**Generosity** to give what I have to others
God's Will to seek and obey the will of God	**Growth** X to keep changing and growing
Health X to be physically well and healthy	**Helpfulness** to be helpful to others
Honesty X to be honest and truthful	**Hope** X to keep a positive and optimistic outlook
Humility to be modest and humble	**Humor** X to see the funny side of life
Independence to be free from dependence on others	**Inner Peace** X to have personal peace
Justice to promote fair and equal treatment for all	**Knowledge** to learn and add to valuable knowledge
Leisure to have time and take time to relax	**Love** X to give and receive love
Loyalty to be loyal and trustworthy	**Moderation** X to avoid excesses and find a middle ground
Nonconformity to question and challenge authority and norms	**Openness** to be open to new things and experiences
Order X to have a well-ordered and organized life	**Passion** to feel strongly and live with intensity

Pleasure to enjoy feeling good	**Popularity** to be well liked by many people
Power to control others and enforce my will	**Purpose** X to have meaning and direction in my life
Rationality to be guided by reason and logic	**Respect** to be treated as a person of worth
Responsibility to make and carry out responsible decisions	**Risk** to take risks and chances
Romance X to have intense, exciting love in my life	**Safety** to be safe and secure
Self-Acceptance to accept myself as I am X	**Self-Discipline** to be disciplined in my own actions
Self-Esteem to feel good about myself X	**Selflessness** to think of others before myself
Self-Knowledge X to have a deep, honest understanding of myself	**Sexuality** to have an active and satisfying sex life
Simplicity to live simply, with the fewest needs	**Skill** to be skilled and masterful
Solitude X to have time and space to be apart from others	**Spirituality** X to live and grow spiritually
Stability X to have a life that stays consistent	**Tolerance** to accept and respect those who differ from me
Tradition to follow respected patterns of the past	**Virtue** to live a morally pure life
Wealth to have plenty of money	**Work** to work hard and well at my life tasks
Other Value	**Other Value**

Most people circle a large number of the values on the list; Alec circled 37, Barbara 42, Colin 32, Dana 39, and Ellie 35. This is typical: many different things are important to us, a state of affairs we become acutely aware of when we feel pulled in more than one direction in the face of even our everyday choices.

Your Companions' Values

Alec

Acceptance, Achievement, Admiration, Adventure, Authenticity, Autonomy, Caring, Challenge, Comfort, Commitment, Confidence, Dependability, Family, Fitness, Forgiveness, Friendship, Fun, Generosity, Health, Helpfulness, Honesty, Hope, Humor, Independence, Leisure, Love, Loyalty, Moderation, Pleasure, Respect, Responsibility, Self-Acceptance, Self-Discipline, Self-Esteem, Skill, Success, Work

Barbara

Acceptance, Achievement, Adventure, Authenticity, Autonomy, Belonging, Caring, Challenge, Commitment, Compassion, Confidence, Contribution, Dependability, Ecology, Excitement, Family, Friendship, Generosity, Growth, Health, Helpfulness, Honesty, Hope, Humility, Humor, Inner Peace, Knowledge, Love, Openness, Passion, Purpose, Respect, Responsibility, Risk, Romance, Self-Esteem, Self-Knowledge, Selflessness, Sexuality, Spirituality, Tolerance, Work

Colin

Acceptance, Admiration, Attractiveness, Authenticity, Autonomy, Caring, Comfort, Compassion, Confidence, Contribution, Creativity, Dependability, Fitness, Forgiveness, Generosity, Health, Honesty, Leisure, Love, Nonconformity, Passion, Pleasure, Respect, Romance, Self-Acceptance, Self-Discipline, Self-Esteem, Sexuality, Skill, Solitude, Tolerance, Work

Dana

Achievement, Authenticity, Belonging, Caring, Commitment, Compassion, Confidence, Contribution, Cooperation, Dependability, Duty, Ecology, Family, Friendship, Fun, Generosity, God's Will, Growth, Health, Helpfulness, Hope, Humility, Independence, Love, Loyalty, Openness, Order, Purpose, Rationality, Respect, Responsibility, Self-Discipline, Self-Esteem, Selflessness, Spirituality, Stability, Tolerance, Tradition, Work

Ellie

Attractiveness, Belonging, Caring, Comfort, Compassion, Confidence, Cooperation, Dependability, Duty, Family, Friendship, Generosity, God's Will, Health, Helpfulness, Honesty, Hope, Humility, Humor, Inner Peace, Justice, Love, Loyalty, Order, Responsibility, Safety, Self-Acceptance, Self-Esteem, Selflessness, Spirituality, Stability, Tolerance, Tradition, Virtue, Work

. . . .

But I want to help you focus on your *core* values, so there is one more step to take: please read through the values you identified as important to you and select the three that are the *most* important to you. Once you've made your selections, I'd like you to think about the values you have chosen. How do you define each of these words for yourself? And what makes each of these values as important as it is to you?

Your companions' chosen values and their responses to these questions appear below.

. . . .

The Values That Matter Most to Me

Alec

Value: *Respect*

How do I define this value?

> Being treated like a person who's worth something because people recognize that you deserve to be treated that way. Being given space to be your own person.

What makes this value so important to me?

> Giving respect and also receiving respect are just important to me—it's hard for me to explain why. You can't really deal with what life throws at you without it.

Value: *Family*

How do I define this value?

> Family are the people in your life that have your back when you need them, and vice versa.

What makes this value so important to me?

> Being a man means making sure your family is taken care of and know-ing that you're there for each other. That's how I was raised, and I'll never believe differently.

Value: *Success*

How do I define this value?

> For me, success means having your work life and your personal life turn out as well as they possibly can. Achieving what you're capable of achieving. Being able to earn a good living, climbing the ladder but making sure that things are right for your family as well.

What makes this value so important to me?

> My father was a success in his work. I looked up to him and wanted to be a success, too. In a way it's how your life is measured, whether you're successful in the things you undertake. That's why I added this one to the list.

Value: *Fitness*

How do I define this value?

> I can't run like I used to, but staying in good shape still matters to me. It's about conditioning and stamina.

What makes this value so important to me?

> Guys who let themselves go get old before their time. I like how I feel when I'm in shape and I need to keep my energy up.

Barbara

Value: *Growth*

How do I define this value?

> Always changing, never becoming stagnant or complacent. Learning, expe-riencing new things, improving, stretching out of your comfort zone. "Chal-lenge" is part of it, too.

What makes this value so important to me?

> Growth feels like a responsibility. We've been given this incredible ability to learn and change. How sad it would be to waste the opportunity to discover what we can be.

Value: *Passion*

How do I define this value?

> To have passion is to have something that grabs you and holds you. It's feeling excited about what you're doing and so committed to it you'd give everything for it.

What makes this value so important to me?

> It has always felt to me like this is what it means to really live and not just go through the motions. As the poet said, if you're not busy living, you're busy dying.

Value: *Caring*

How do I define this value?

> Reaching down inside yourself and giving to others in your life and in the world in a full way. It requires thoughtfulness, generosity, and humility.

What makes this value so important to me?

> I was raised to believe that we are responsible to others as well as ourselves. It is a value that Steve and I share—really, it's what drew me to him, and it's one of the things that has held us together all these years.

Colin

Value: *Authenticity*

How do I define this value?

> Being true to yourself, yes, but also knowing who you are, what you really think and feel. And not being afraid of letting others see who you are. Being real, not pretending or portraying yourself as something you're not.

What makes this value so important to me?

> When you lose touch with yourself, your life is set adrift. It's also a question of trust. If you are not authentic, then how can I trust what you say? If I am not authentic, then how can you trust me?

Value: *Creativity*

How do I define this value?

> It's so much more than having original ideas and making new things. It's expression of your Self, your vision, your inner struggles, sparks, and inspirations. It's bringing all that's unique in you out into the world.

What makes this value so important to me?

> This is so much a part of who I am, I would not know how to be otherwise. It's what gives me the greatest sense of well-being—when I am being creative, everything else goes away and I'm who I'm supposed to be.

Value: *Compassion*

How do I define this value?

> Not judging others narrowly. There's usually more to people than meets the eye. I think compassion develops when you think outside the box about others and are then able to feel more appreciative and caring toward them.

What makes this value so important to me?

> I have felt what it's like to be pigeonholed. And I have done my share of judging, too. Looking at the whole person, his struggles and circumstances, before deciding who he is makes me feel on the side of the angels.

Dana

Value: *Contribution*

How do I define this value?

> Not just adding "something" to the world but something that improves the lives of others. Leaving something behind that makes a difference to vulnerable people.

What makes this value so important to me?

> It gives me a sense of purpose, which I almost chose as one of my top values. But the purpose is to give back, because I know I've been given so much.

Value: *Dependability*

How do I define this value?

> People should be able to count on you to be there for them when they need you. Also, they should be able to trust that you will always try to show up to do your best.

What makes this value so important to me?

> I pride myself on being this way. I am dependable, and I respect others who are as well. This is what children need most from the adults in their lives.

Value: *Spirituality*

How do I define this value?

> Spirituality means paying attention to your awareness of the preciousness of life and being guided by your deepest beliefs, faith, and care for humanity, no matter what your religion is or what your idea of God is.

What makes this value so important to me?

> This is my deepest value and the part of me that keeps my life on track. No one can guide me the way this does. This is the wellspring from where my love, respect, determination, stability, and self-awareness all emerge.

Ellie

Value: *Family*

How do I define this value?

> Family are the people you love and cherish, who make your house a home, your world a welcoming place, and your life worth living. They are the people you would do anything for and who would do anything for you.

What makes this value so important to me?

> Without my family I'd have nothing, and nothing I have would matter.

Value: *God's Will*

How do I define this value?

> I think of this as working to learn and follow what God wants for you to do on this earth. To be the best person you can be while you're here and do the best for others that you can.

What makes this value so important to me?

> I have been blessed with many gifts in my life. If I'm not grateful enough to live that life according to His will, then that's a problem.

Value: *Self-Esteem*

How do I define this value?

> Loving yourself. Feeling good about who you are and trying to improve in whatever way you can. Doing what you believe is right so that you can be proud of yourself.

What makes this value so important to me?

> *I laughed after I chose this, because I realized that I was just writing about how I didn't have self-esteem. But I see it in my clients. When something boosts their self-esteem, they get a burst of energy—and watch out!*

Now it's your turn. Please ask yourself: "Which three values are the *most* important to me?" (You may find it challenging to limit yourself to just three, but the goal is to think seriously about which of your values really matter to you the most. If you must include a fourth, or even a fifth, to do justice to what you really care about, of course you should do so.) "How do I define each of these words for myself?" (The short definitions I provided may or may not match what the words mean to you personally.) And "What makes each of these values as important as it is to me?" Use your journal to enter your answers or use the form at *www.guilford.com/zuckoff-forms*.

What Role Do Your Values Play in Your Life?

As you've been writing about the core values you identified, you've probably found yourself thinking about ways those values shape the way you live and the choices you make; you may even have begun to write about those things. I'd like you to focus on those thoughts in more detail by describing the ways you are already living out the values you hold most dear.

Your companions' responses appear below.

How Am I Already Living Out the Values That Matter Most to Me?

Alec

Values: Respect, Family, Success, Fitness

> *I've put a lot of energy into succeeding, for myself but also for my family. I know I could get that promotion if I went for it because my boss recognizes that. At the same time, even though Wendy hasn't been happy with me being away so much, when my family needs me, they know I'm there. As for respect, I always treat my coworkers with the respect they deserve. We had a new hire, and I could tell he was pretty green. Some of the other guys were treating him that way, and I didn't like it. So I started buddying up and*

talking to him. Not like I would to a kid, but like an equal, as a young guy who had something to offer. That guy treats me with great respect now, because I gave it to him. And I respect Wendy, too. When these other guys, even the married ones, are hitting on some waitress, I'm heading home. Fitness, well, I've been slacking off on that lately.

Barbara

Values: Growth, Passion, Caring

I have grown through the challenges I've taken up with my children. I have pushed myself past my comfort zone in many ways. It would not matter how tired, busy, or under the weather I felt, if the school needed a volunteer, I was there. I wanted to grow along with them. Caring is just how I always am. One of my friends called me recently to see if I'd come over to help her with her kids because everyone in the house had the flu. She couldn't stop vomiting, and her husband and kids were doing the same. It was right before we were taking a trip to attend my niece's wedding. My husband was worried I would bring their illness with me, but we both agreed that I had to go and help.

Colin

Values: Authenticity, Creativity, Compassion

Authenticity is closely related to integrity for me. It's about being true to yourself and not hiding who you are. One of our close friends even mentioned that he has a great deal of respect for that, and that Paul is lucky to have someone in his life who works so hard to be true to himself and wants the same for him. The one place where I was failing, ironically, was in trying to pretend to myself that I was perfectly willing to try to control my anger with Paul and had no mixed feelings about it. Owning how I really feel about all this is much more authentic. My creativity shows up everywhere: in my work, in my home. People remark on our place from the minute they walk in; I have a very strong design sense, and I have to live in an environment that is aesthetically pleasing. I offer my creativity to friends, too—I enjoy consulting for them on their homes. Compassion is something I've developed slowly over the years. Trying to see what others' challenges are helps me when I am confronted with people who are homophobic. It still makes me angry, but it doesn't eat me up anymore, and sometimes I'm able to wonder about how they got that way. A couple of times I was even able to talk to the person in a way that got him thinking. That felt like a personal triumph!

Dana

Values: *Contribution, Dependability, Spirituality*

> I used to feel I was contributing at my job, but I don't feel that much now. The contribution I make now is to my family, and it does make a big difference for them. I'm very dependable that way. I am dependable even when it's not going to be noticed. Last week I was out with friends, and I said I had to go because I needed to be up early to cover for a coworker. When I added, "Not that anyone would notice even if I didn't," my friends gave me a hard time about leaving, but I told them that all that matters is that I would know. My spirituality—it's with me every moment of every day. It guides me. It shows up in how I respond to others' adversities. Whenever there is an opportunity to be kind to someone, I am. It is as simple as listening to an older person on the bus who wants to talk about her life, and who might be lonely or scared.

Ellie

Values: *Family, God's Will, Self-Esteem*

> I live out my values of family and God's will daily. I am not perfect at it, of course, but I think about my family's well-being all the time. I think about what I'll cook for them, I watch out for their health and their doctor appointments, I try to keep a clean home. I also try to support each of them, including Gil, to follow their dreams. Last month he told me he wanted to start making furniture again. He wanted to have a shop in the house when we first moved here and the kids were little, but it wasn't practical because of the space. But this time I decided to surprise him, for his birthday. I asked the kids to help me clean out the garage while he was away, and I bought a small sanding tool and wrapped it with the instruction to go into the garage. He was so thrilled! He's been setting up equipment, and I can hardly wait to see him doing what he loves again. I believe that by trying to be the best wife and mother I can be I am following God's will for me. As for self-esteem, I'm really good at building that up in others. I always look for the best in everyone—my clients and my friends, and all my family.

Now it's your turn. Please ask yourself: "How would someone who was observing me as I go about my life know that these are my values?" Be specific and give as many examples as you can think of. Because I want you to focus first on what you feel good about in how you're living your life, if you find yourself also thinking about ways you're not living out your values as much as you would like, please set those thoughts aside for now. If that's true of one or two of your values in particular, just write about the value or values that your life exemplifies. Use your journal or the form at *www.guilford.com/zuckoff-forms* to record your answers.

As we saw in the stories of Bonnie and John, and noted previously, when people begin to think seriously about their values they often realize they would like to be living out one or more of them more fully than they have been. If they've been stuck in ambivalence about an important area of their life, it's even more likely that two or more of their core values are in conflict or that influences other than their values have been shaping their choices. These influences might include everyday rewards of the behavior they're thinking about changing, costs they think change might bring, or fears about what trying to change might mean.

This is what I'd like you to think about now—how you would like to be living out one or more of your most important values more fully and what is keeping you from doing so. In particular, what role might your current behavior or situation be playing?

Your companions' thoughts about these questions appear below.

How Would I Like to Be Living Out My Core Values More Fully? How Is My Current Behavior or Situation Keeping Me from Doing That?

Alec

Values: Respect, Family, Success, Fitness

I definitely want to get back to taking care of myself physically. I know how to do that; it's just a matter of making the time. Before, I would have said that Wendy is trying to get me to stop doing what I need to do to succeed, so family was getting in the way of success. But now I'm thinking that maybe it's the other way around. Maybe my competitive fire got me carried away. Work is always going to be demanding, and I'll always want to excel, so I'm not about to relax. But I've been so focused on winning I haven't been putting much effort into my marriage or Jen. Or much of anything else, either—like our friends. I lost that balance, and I need to get it back. And I guess somehow I knew it, and that's why I kept putting off asking for that bigger district—it would have magnified the whole scenario. So at least that makes sense now. I still want Wendy to appreciate how I take care of her and Jen financially, but I guess I haven't been making it easy for her to do that. Which is where the respect thing comes in, I guess. I've been pretty hyped about Wendy not respecting me when I come home late and she nags me about my drinking. I still don't like it, but I have to admit that I wasn't thinking about how respectfully I've been treating her. Brushing her off—anyone would be unhappy about that. Staying out later than I have to isn't going to make anything better either. I think it would be good to get back to more of the respect that we used to show each other.

Barbara

Values: Growth, Passion, Caring

For so long my passion was my children. When our last child left, I began to remember the sexual part of me that I'd set aside for years and wanted to feel that way again. I couldn't imagine having that with Steve, so I started thinking about other men. And then all my feelings of care and commitment made that seem impossible and my guilt and panic took over. I do need to feel passionate again. But it surprised me to remember how close Steve and I were when we were first together and to realize how strong the value of caring was in pulling us together. It felt like reconnecting a little. And of course he always encouraged and supported me to take on all the challenges I wanted to throw myself into. So maybe I haven't been fair to him? It's been so long since we've spent real time together that didn't revolve around the kids, maybe we both forgot what we had once, and maybe there's more to explore there. And maybe I also need another outlet for growth. Maybe I've been too quick to dismiss thoughts about working again and finding new challenges in the wider world.

Colin

Values: Authenticity, Creativity, Compassion

As immersed as I am in being creative, I haven't been creative at all in dealing with this situation. I've actually been very noncreative, even rigid. Using my art to help me work through complex feelings and discover new ways of looking at things is usually like breathing for me, but somehow I lost sight of that. And what's ironic is that that's the most authentic way I can be. So stubbornness and treating Paul like the enemy has kept me from being my best self. And forget about compassion. I've been more compassionate to homophobes than to my life partner. I haven't really tried to understand what this has been all about for him, not in a deep way. So my answer is, I have my work cut out for me.

Dana

Values: Contribution, Dependability, Spirituality

By becoming a teacher. Honestly, I know that's how I can make my best contribution. As much as I love my family, I don't feel good about being so dependable for them at the expense of making a larger contribution. I have been spending a lot of time looking at this practically and worrying about the financial aspects and my responsibilities to the people in my life, but not what I was put on earth to accomplish, in addition to being a dependable, loving daughter. In other words, I haven't been treating my spirituality as being as important as it should be. It's funny, because if it weren't for my family I wouldn't have these values in the first place.

Ellie

Values: *Family, God's Will, Self-Esteem*

> *I don't really believe it's selfish to take care of myself or even let my family take care of me. I'm part of my family, too! But I <u>feel</u> wrong about it. I don't believe it's God's will that I turn away support or get down on myself. I don't think God expects me to be a saint. I think He wants me to love myself, like He loves me. I just have a major block in me that stops me from doing nice things for myself or accepting it when other people want to help me, even though I know that taking better care of myself is good for them and not just me.*

Now it's your turn. Please ask yourself, "Is there a conflict between my values that might be contributing to keeping me stuck? Are there ways I am acting that are in tension with one or more of my values, keeping me from living them out as fully as I would wish?" Record your answers in your journal or use the form at *www.guilford.com/zuckoff-forms*.

Finally, I'd like you to focus now on what it would take for you to live out your core values more fully. First, consider your companions' responses, shown below.

What Changes Would I Have to Make to Live Out My Values More Fully?

Alec

Values: *Respect, Family, Success, Fitness*

> *I would need to figure out how to make more time for Wendy and Jen and our friends, for that matter. Also for myself, to start working out again, and maybe even to get out to the garage to work on my Camaro—it's been gathering dust for longer than I like to think about. I guess that's what getting some balance back would mean. I'd also have to be more respectful toward Wendy when I come home and figure out how to get her to be more respectful toward me. Cutting down on my drinking with my customers would help with that.*

Barbara

Values: *Growth, Passion, Caring*

> *I might have to rethink what I think I know about Steve. It's been a long time since I let myself see him as more than a provider and companion. He is*

that, but I haven't considered in years whether he could be more than that. I would also have to take a chance and be more open with him and see if we could get to know each other again, in a deeper way. It's scary to think about because I honestly don't know what I would find. Someone who I could feel passion with? Or a good man who is who he is and is satisfied with that? And I also might have to start thinking about what kind of work I can do, what kind I want to do, and even let myself imagine what it would be like to relaunch a career for myself.

Colin

Values: Authenticity, Creativity, Compassion

Be more creative in how I can learn to express my anger differently and more compassionate with Paul about how hard this has been for him and how my anger affects him.

Dana

Values: Contribution, Dependability, Spirituality

I would have to get up the courage to talk with my family about my true feelings and what I want to do. I would have to decide that I am willing to risk letting my family down to do what I feel called to do. It feels like I would be taking myself more seriously and letting my spirituality guide me more fully.

Ellie

Values: Family, God's Will, Self-Esteem

I'd have to get better at treating what I want as important. Like losing weight. Funny how I've hardly been thinking about that. But it <u>is</u> important to me, and I know it would help my self-esteem. It's just that I would have to be able to do that without neglecting Gil and the kids. And learn to let them help me more. Even though I think they'd be willing, I'm not so sure that any of us would know how to do that!

Now it's your turn. Ask yourself: "What would I have to do to live out those values more fully in the future? What changes, if any, would I need to make in the behavior or situation I have been working on? What would I need, or what might help me, live out those values more fully than I already am?" Record your thoughts in your journal or use the form at *www.guilford. com/zuckoff-forms.*

Reflecting on Your Values Exploration

I'd like to invite you now to reflect on your understanding of the values you hold most dear, their place in your life, and their relationship to your dilemma. Please reread your responses to the first three activities in this chapter. Then read your response to the fourth activity, "What Changes Would I Have to Make to Live Out My Values More Fully?" out loud, listening to yourself as you read. Then ask yourself, "Where does this leave me now?" Read your companions' reflections before recording your answer in your journal or using the form "Reflecting on My Values Exploration" at *www.guilford.com/zuckoff-forms*. Once you've written your reflection, please read *it* out loud as well.

Here are your companions' reflections:

- *Alec:* "It looks like it's pretty clear what I need to do. Putting work and family back in balance and carving out some time to get myself into better shape, too. Not because anyone is telling me to but because I can see that I got off track a little and I want to get back on track. Drinking less just makes sense as part of all that."

- *Barbara:* "I don't know how I let my focus get so narrow, but I'm feeling differently as my perspective has widened. Not knowing what the future holds but thinking about trying to create something new with Steve and exploring a career restart after all these years is giving me that old pit-of-the-stomach feeling that tells me I'm on to something."

- *Colin:* "I'm ready to work on this for real now."

- *Dana:* "Getting more in touch with my spiritual side helps me see things more clearly. If I decide to do what I love, my family will be behind me—maybe not right away, but in time they will understand. I have been worrying about their initial reaction, but I know they want me to be fulfilled and to do what matters in my life. I'm excited to get started."

- *Ellie:* "Reminding myself that losing weight would be good for my family and not just me helps me feel less bad about letting them help me if that's what I need to be able to lose weight. Which I think it is. I'll just have to make sure I'm not taking anything away from them. If I can do that, I might even develop some self-esteem!"

THE WAY FORWARD

The chapters in Part II were designed to help you resolve your ambivalence by exploring your importance and confidence for change and the implications of your core values for the decision you have been trying to make. If the activities you've completed have had their intended effect, you've begun to see a path out of the dilemma you've been stuck in opening up before you. Are you ready to take that path?

● ● ● ● ● ● ● ● ● ●

Second Interlude
Ready or Not?

It's time to decide whether the work you've done has left you ready to commit to a direction forward. To help with that decision (or to help strengthen your resolve if you've already decided), I'd like you to look back and think about where you started, where you are now, and how you've gotten here. Please go all the way back to your response to the first activity I asked you to complete—to tell "the story of your ambivalence"—and reread all of your responses right up to your last reflection. Then ask yourself: "How was I thinking about my situation when I began? How has my perspective on it changed, and how am I seeing it now?" But first, consider your companions' responses, shown below.

. . . .

A Look Back

Alec

How did I see things at the start?

> *I saw this as my wife's problem. I thought she was being pretty unreasonable, and I was trying to figure out how to get her to knock it off. I didn't really feel like I needed to change anything.*

How do I see things now?

> *Changes need to be made. It's not about "having a problem"—it's wanting things to be better and figuring out how to make them better in one area without harming another area. I don't think it has to be a big deal.*

Barbara

How did I see things at the start?

> I felt trapped—either I hurt Steve and the kids so I can have a life or I stay and spend my life feeling miserable. And I felt as though I had to decide immediately and just live with the decision. I felt guilty and desperate because I couldn't decide.

How do I see things now?

> I am hopeful. I have other choices than to sacrifice myself or my marriage. I have a scared/excited feeling that I recognize from all the times I jumped feet-first into uncharted territory and hit the ground running. I haven't felt that in a long time.

Colin

How did I see things at the start?

> I was divided inside, but I didn't know it, or really I didn't want to know it. Part of me wanted to do what Paul was asking, but part of me resented him for asking it and felt blamed. I was also starting to have a sense of futility, not being able to get a handle on my anger, even though I didn't want to admit that either.

How do I see things now?

> I'm not conflicted about changing. I know what I want and what matters to me. I'm looking at this more as a challenge, to come up with more creative ways of managing my anger and get better at talking with Paul about why some things upset me and how we can be better together.

Dana

How did I see things at the start?

> I was seeing this as an issue of responsibility. I felt it would be immature to do what I wanted instead of what was practical. I was really focused on finances and helping my family.

How do I see things now?

> As part of my spiritual development. Becoming a teacher would be serving the greater good and fulfilling my potential. It's a good decision.

Ellie

How did I see things at the start?

> I was feeling very hopeless because I had failed so many times. And I was feeling pretty bad about myself. I really wasn't even sure why I bothered to pick up this book. I guess I just couldn't let myself give up.

How do I see things now?

> I don't feel hopeless. I'm still not sure I can do this, though. I want to be nicer to myself, and I think I want to let my family help me more, especially Gil. It's not selfish to do that because it makes him feel good to support me, and if I lose weight it will be good for everyone, not just me.

. . . .

Now it's your turn. Write your answers in your journal or use the form at *www.guilford.com/zuckoff-forms*.

RECOGNIZING READINESS

It's important to be genuinely ready to change before going on to the activities in the third section of this book. This doesn't mean that you should expect to feel 100% sure that you've made the right decision; in fact, many people who embark on a process of change continue to harbor at least a little bit of doubt or trepidation at the prospect of launching themselves into the unknown. However, it does mean that you should feel confident in your decision and willing to do what it takes to carry it out.

Being ready to change means being wholehearted even if you're less than completely sure.

How to judge whether you're ready? Sometimes it's an easy call—you feel a growing sense of eagerness as you think concretely about taking the next step, even if you feel nervous about some aspects of what you're about to do. But things are not always quite so clear-cut—you may think you know what your next step is, but you may not be sure how it's going to work out or whether you've found the right solution; or, you're not so much eager to change as you've come to see change as a necessity.

So I'd like you to ask yourself how ready you are to change. If you don't feel sure yet that you will be *able* to do what you have in mind, remember that I haven't yet helped you develop a plan for change, so not knowing how it will work is to be expected.

Ask yourself these questions:

- "How ready am I right now to commit to developing a plan for carrying out the decision I've made and, once I feel confident in my plan, following it to make change happen?"
- "How would I describe the way I'm feeling about change right now?"

. . . .

Readiness to Change

How **ready** am I *right now* to develop and carry out a plan for change?

0	1	2	3	4	5	6	7	8	9	10
Not at all					Moderately					Extremely

. . . .

Here are your companions' responses to consider before you write yours:

- Alec chose an **8**: "I know I need to do this, and I don't think I'll have too much trouble pulling it off. I like thinking about how it will be when things are back in balance and Wendy and I are on the same side again."
- Barbara chose a **9**: "After so much time in turmoil it's a relief to know what I'm going to do, even though I'm also nervous and I don't know how it will turn out. There's a possibility it could be really good, which is exciting. I'm eager and curious, and I have been thinking about possible ways to start."
- Colin chose an **8**: "I'm ready to start planning. I know how I want things to be between Paul and me, and now I need to put my creativity to work to figure out how we can do it. This needs to happen because I do not want to lose him."
- Dana chose a **10**: "It's time for me to talk with my family about what I want to do. I've already begun to look into information on the different schools and their financial assistance programs. This feels right. I'm not doubting myself now."
- Ellie chose a **5**: "I feel a lot more ready than I did before. I feel different, in a good way. But also really anxious when I think about actually doing it. Maybe it's just hard to believe that this time will

turn out different than all the other times I tried. The first steps, like talking with my family, feel pretty scary."

Either on the rating scale on page 165 or using the one at *www.guilford. com/zuckoff-forms*, circle the number that represents your readiness. Then, in your journal or on the online form, answer the questions above.

Perhaps the number you chose is all you need to tell you what's next for you. But a good way to confirm just how ready you are is to look for *mobilizing change talk* in what you wrote. You may remember from the First Interlude that, unlike preparatory talk, which builds importance and confidence for changing or keeping things the same, mobilizing talk expresses *intentions* and gets people "mobilized" to take action. As we discussed earlier, when people are engaging in mobilizing change talk, you'll hear phrases like these expressing:

- *Commitment*: "I will . . .", "I'm going to . . .", "I promise to . . ."
- *Activation*: "I'm ready to . . .", "I'm willing to . . .", "I'm prepared to . . ."
- *Taking steps*: "I started to . . .", "I'm trying to . . .", "I've begun to . . ."

You may also hear phrases like these expressing:

- *Positive feelings*: "I'm excited about . . .", "I'm eager to . . .", "I can't wait to . . ."
- *Resolve*: "I've decided to . . .", "Nothing will keep me from . . .", "It's time to . . ."
- *Envisioning change*: "When I think of what it will be like . . .", "Imagine how . . ."

Do you see phrases like these in your last response?

THE WAY FORWARD

Ready to Change

If, like Alec, Barbara, Colin, and Dana, you chose a number between 7 and 10 and engaged in mobilizing change talk, you are ready to begin planning for change. Although 10 might express a higher level of certainty or enthusiasm than 7, there are various reasons why a person might be at either the top or the bottom of that range and still be "ready enough" to move ahead. Please go on to Part III.

Not Ready to Change

If you chose a number between 0 and 3, it's likely that your response included little or no mobilizing change talk and at least some mobilizing sustain talk—that is, expressions of commitment, resolve, or steps toward keeping things the way they are as well as negative feelings about change.

You might have chosen that number because you've realized that change is not the right decision for you. If you feel confident that whatever you might gain by making a change is outweighed by what you would lose, or you simply feel satisfied with the status quo, then you have resolved your ambivalence. There's no reason for you to go on to Part III.

On the other hand, if you feel as though you should try to change, even though you're reluctant, you might be considering going on despite not being ready. I would recommend that you *not* go on to Part III under these circumstances. *Halfhearted action*—embarking on change without feeling committed or ready—follows a fairly predictable course for most people. There's a high risk that their efforts to change will falter because they don't feel willing to make change a high priority, they don't bring the full weight of their creativity and resourcefulness to bear, and they aren't determined enough to push through any obstacles that might arise. As they find themselves struggling, they're apt to become discouraged and start wondering whether the change is worth it or whether they really have a chance of making it happen. They may also begin to resent "having" to do something when their heart isn't in it.

If this description sounds familiar, it could be because Colin was engaging in halfhearted action at the start of this book. Unless people engaging in halfhearted action are able to come to see their situation in a different way (as Colin did), it's a short distance to giving up—feeling disappointed and less confident at best, and at worst, creating or reinforcing the sense that they're helpless to make change happen, with all the negative consequences that outlook brings (self-criticism, hopelessness, or resignation to an unhappy state of affairs). Worst of all, when an attempt ends this way, it makes it harder for the person to feel ready, willing, and able to change in the future.

> Halfhearted attempts to change not only end in disappointment—they can poison the well of motivation for future attempts.

Instead, I encourage you to consider other resources for helping people resolve ambivalence and move forward in their lives. If the spirit and practices of MI feel like a good fit for you, even though you've not made as much progress as you may have hoped, then seeking out a counselor who practices MI and works with people who are dealing with issues like yours could be a solution. More generally, practitioners who specialize in the issue you are struggling with may be able to help in a way that a self-guided approach like this one could not. The most important thing to take away from your experience in working on your ambivalence with this book is that no source of help works for everyone, because everyone is different. There is every reason to believe you will find a solution to your dilemma elsewhere if you have not found it here.

Leaning Toward Change

Finally, if, like Ellie, you chose a number between 4 and 6, you're most likely leaning toward change but not quite ready. I'd like to see if I can help you feel more resolved.

One effect of ambivalence is that it can make it hard to see the forest for the trees. Mentally surrounded by competing thoughts and feelings—reasons to change and reasons not to; wanting a change and also dreading it; hopes for success and fears of failure; anxiety, guilt, curiosity, anticipation—it's easy to lose sight of what you're doing all this for.

So now I'd like to help you take a step back and see the big picture. Imagine that you decided to make the change you're considering, and 6 months or a year later everything has gone just as you hoped it would. Surveying your life as it would be then, please ask yourself these questions:

- "How do I know that I've succeeded? How is my life different? What am I doing, how am I feeling, and what do others notice about me?"
- "In hindsight, what is the best thing about having made the change, and what would have been the worst thing about not having made it?"

Consider Ellie's response, shown on the next page, before writing your own.

Imagining Change

Ellie

How do I know that I've succeeded? How is my life different? What am I doing, how am I feeling, and what do others notice about me? What is the best thing about having made this change? What would have been the worst thing about not having made it?

> *That's pretty hard to imagine. I'm thinner and healthier. More energy—I don't get as tired as fast, which is nice because it's hard to keep up with everything when you wear out so quickly. I imagine getting dressed in the morning and feeling good about how I look instead of disgusted. I go out more with my kids instead of making excuses not to. Shopping with my friends sometimes. Gil and I are more intimate. People probably notice that I seem more relaxed and happy. I feel happier—that's the best thing. If I didn't make this change, well, I'd still be feeling like I do now, missing out and letting myself and everyone else in my life down.*

Now it's your turn. Write your answers to the questions in your journal or in the form at *www.guilford.com/zuckoff-forms*. Once you've written your response, please listen to yourself as you read it aloud.

Having imagined the effects of succeeding at change, how has that affected how ready you feel to undertake it now, if at all? Here's Ellie's response:

> "Right now, just thinking about it this way, it moves me up at least to a 5 or 6. I wish it would stay there. I think it would if doing it didn't make me so anxious."

Now write your own answer in your journal or use the form at *www.guilford.com/zuckoff-forms*.

If you found that imagining having changed feels good, then your doubts about committing to change could be related to something specific, but as-yet unidentified, about the prospect of the change that is creating discomfort. This is especially likely if, like Ellie, you've tried repeatedly to make this change without success, although it's also possible that the source of that discomfort has kept you from trying to change until now.

I want to be clear that I am not talking about "fear of success," "self-sabotage," "wanting" to fail, or not feeling worthy of doing better or having what you want; those kinds of "self-defeating" motivations are quite uncommon, despite what you may have heard. What I mean is that, as much as you might want to make the change you're considering, and as valuable as its benefits might be, there might also be a *cost* that you're vaguely aware of but have not yet put into words here, which may be holding you back.

To see whether this is true for you, please ask yourself this: "What might change cost me? If I let myself imagine working on change, what discomfort, if any, do I feel?"

Consider Ellie's response, shown below, before you write yours in your journal or in the form at *www.guilford.com/zuckoff-forms.*

. . . .

What Might Change Cost Me?

Ellie

> Besides feeling uncomfortable about asking my family for help, to be honest I've been thinking about having to give up my comfort foods. They get me through my stressful days. And giving them up not just while I'm dieting, but forever? That's pretty hard for me to imagine. And that means that even if I drop a few pounds I can't see how I'm going to be able to keep them off. But if I can't, then why bother?

. . . .

Ellie identified something she's not sure she's ready to give up in making the change she wants to make. Perhaps this reservation has been there at other times when Ellie started to diet, and it's one of the reasons losing weight has been so hard for her for so long. If you've identified something similar, the first thing I want to point out is that you have actually been doing a kind of "envisioning" of change. That is, you are imagining what change would be like and bumping up against something that pulls you up short.

The solution to this problem is *not* to try to ignore or talk yourself out of whatever it is that feels important to hold on to. Why? Because to do that would be yet another way of pressuring yourself to change, and after all the good work you've done to set that pressure aside and give yourself a good listening-to, it would be a shame to let that happen now.

Here's how I'd suggest approaching it instead. The behavior or object you're reluctant to let go of is a way of meeting a real and legitimate need, and that need is not likely to go away. To feel ready to change, you will either have to find a way to keep what you have without its interfering with the change you want to make or replace what you are giving up so that you can meet that need in another way.

So please ask yourself these two sets of questions:

- "Do I have a need that is being met by what I'm reluctant to let go of? If so, what is that need?"
- "Is there a way to hold on to that behavior or object and still succeed at change? If not, is it possible to find another way to meet that need that would fit with and support the decision about change I'm leaning toward making?"

Consider Ellie's response to these questions, shown in the table below, before you write yours in your journal or in the form at *www.guilford.com/ zuckoff-forms.*

. . . .

The Need Being Met by the Status Quo

Ellie

What need, if any, is what I am holding on to meeting?

> My comfort foods really do comfort me. They're my stress relievers and little rewards at the end of the day, when I'm tired and in the kitchen making dinner for everyone and then later when I finally have a little quiet time to myself. They keep me company and give me a break and make me feel good, and I can always count on them doing that for me.

Can I hold on to it and succeed at change? Could there be another way to meet that need?

> I guess I could try cutting down instead of cutting them out. But I don't know if that would work because they're all high fat and high calorie, which is what makes them so comforting. Plus, I don't know how I would feel about having to restrict myself—it might take some of the pleasure away if I had to count the cookies I eat. I think the other idea would work better if I could think of something. I didn't really think before about other kinds of rewards and comforts.

. . . .

It would be unrealistic to expect you to have come up just now with a definitive replacement for a long-standing way of meeting an important need, and that was not the purpose of the activity. Instead, I hope that realizing there's a good reason you've felt hesitant to commit to change, and that succeeding at change would involve taking care of that need and not trying to ignore it or persuade yourself that it doesn't matter, might help you feel a bit more optimistic about being able to make change happen. And it's important to know that, if you do choose to move ahead, making sure your needs are met will be one of the guiding principles of the planning process I will lead you through.

So at this point, if I asked you once more to rate how ready you are on that 0–10 scale to develop and carry out a plan for change, what number would you choose and why?

- -

Readiness Redux for the Second Interlude

How **ready** am I *right now* to develop and carry out a plan for change?

0	1	2	3	4	5	6	7	8	9	10
Not at all					Moderately					Extremely

- -

Ellie chooses a 7:

> "I owe it to myself to try one more time. I know it won't be easy, but it's worth it to me if there's even a decent chance that I'll finally be able to look the way I want to look and feel how I want to feel."

How about you? Please circle the number that represents your readiness now, using the rating scale above or the form "Readiness Redux for the Second Interlude" at *www.guilford.com/zuckoff-forms*. If you've chosen at least a 7, please go on to Part III. If you're still leaning but not yet there, consider returning to the activities in Chapters 4 and 5, which may draw out different thoughts and feelings in the aftermath of your reflections on your values in Chapter 6. Although I cannot guarantee it, I am hopeful that the work you have been doing will be rewarded.

Finding YOUR Way to Change

Third Interlude
Planning for Change

When he was very young, our son enjoyed listening to a recording of the traditional children's song "There's a Hole in My Bucket." Do you remember how it goes? It takes the form of a conversation between "Henry," who has the problem named in the title, and "Liza," the practical-minded girl Henry addresses.

> There's a hole in my bucket, dear Liza, dear Liza,
> There's a hole in my bucket, dear Liza, a hole.
> Then mend it, dear Henry, dear Henry, dear Henry,
> Then mend it, dear Henry, dear Henry, mend it.

Liza thinks Henry is asking her what he should do about his situation, and her response is to offer him advice. This does not resolve the situation, though. Henry wants more detail on how this whole bucket-mending thing works, and Liza is happy to provide it:

> With what shall I mend it, dear Liza, dear Liza,
> With what shall I mend it, dear Liza, with what?
> With a straw, dear Henry, dear Henry, dear Henry,
> With a straw, dear Henry, dear Henry, a straw.

Now, you might expect that Henry would take Liza's advice and go off to fix his bucket. However, Henry has more questions:

> *If the straw be too long, dear Liza, dear Liza,*
> *If the straw be too long, dear Liza, too long?*
> *Then cut it, dear Henry, dear Henry, dear Henry,*
> *Then cut it, dear Henry, dear Henry, cut it.*
> *With what shall I cut it, dear Liza, dear Liza,*
> *With what shall I cut it, dear Liza, with what?*

Uh-oh. Liza has probably begun to realize that, the more advice she offers, the more questions Henry asks—in fact, the more helpless he seems to be.

> *With a knife, dear Henry, dear Henry, dear Henry,*
> *With a knife, dear Henry, dear Henry, a knife.*
> *If the knife be too dull, dear Liza, dear Liza,*
> *If the knife be too dull, dear Liza, too dull?*
> *Then sharpen it, dear Henry, dear Henry, dear Henry,*
> *Then sharpen it, dear Henry, dear Henry, sharpen it.*
> *With what shall I sharpen it, dear Liza, dear Liza,*
> *With what shall I sharpen it, dear Liza, with what?*

By this point it is surely clear to Liza—and maybe to Henry—that things have taken an unhelpful turn. In the recording our son listened to over and over, Liza's growing exasperation with Henry comes across clearly in her tone of voice and the sighs that punctuate her responses; as the song wends its way painfully to its end, she literally begins to *moan* each time her answer begets yet another question.

> *With a stone, dear Henry, dear Henry, dear Henry,*
> *With a stone, dear Henry, dear Henry, a stone.*
> *If the stone is too rough, dear Liza, dear Liza,*
> *If the stone is too rough, dear Liza, too rough?*
> *Then wet it, dear Henry, dear Henry, dear Henry,*
> *Then wet it, dear Henry, dear Henry, wet it.*
> *With what shall I wet it, dear Liza, dear Liza,*
> *With what shall I wet it, dear Liza, with what?*
> *With water, dear Henry, dear Henry, dear Henry,*
> *With water, dear Henry, dear Henry, with water.*
> *And how shall I fetch it, dear Liza, dear Liza,*
> *And how shall I fetch it, dear Liza, and how?*

As the song approaches its inevitable conclusion, even Liza seems, with dawning horror, to see what's coming. Yet she is powerless to stop it, trapped in the role she has taken on.

> *In a bucket, dear Henry, dear Henry, dear Henry,*
> *In a bucket, dear Henry, dear Henry, your bucket.*
> *There's a hole in my bucket, dear Liza, dear Liza,*
> *There's a hole in my bucket, dear Liza, a hole.*

With this, Liza lets out a shriek, and the recording comes crashing to an end. Three things are unmistakable: the conversation we have just heard has been an exercise in futility; Liza will dread any future installment; and Henry is no further along in solving his problem than when he started, despite Liza's good intentions.

What relevant lessons for your situation can we draw from this old song? Contrary to the usual interpretation—that Henry is a bit of a dolt, and poor Liza's patience with him is sorely tested—I would argue that Liza's assumption that Henry wants and expects to be told what to do, and that her job is to tell him, sets the entire, unproductive conversation in motion. (Surely Henry did not need Liza to tell him to mend something he knew was broken?) In fact, "There's a Hole in My Bucket" provides an excellent illustration of what can happen when a person who has decided that there is a problem to be fixed or a change that needs to be made is offered "help" in the form of all-purpose, one-size-fits-all advice. Leaping immediately into the mode of "expert," Liza has in fact helped to create the nightmarish scenario in which she finds herself.

So let's consider an alternate scenario. What if, after the failure of her initial attempt to help, Liza had tried to draw out Henry's ideas about how to solve the problem? She might have discovered that Henry had his own resources to draw on and that his thoughts about what kind of approach seemed workable to him were a better guide for coming up with a plan than her suggestions. She might also have recognized that his increasing passivity in response to her advice—"With what shall I wet it?"—was a product of her taking over and telling him what to do; she might even have wondered whether he simply fell into an exaggerated version of the role she had prepared for him: a person who cannot be expected to think for himself or act on his own.

At this point the analogy may itself be in danger of springing a leak. But if this account holds water (sorry, couldn't resist), it has important implications for how I can be most helpful to your efforts to develop an effective plan for change.

HOW CAN I HELP YOU PLAN FOR CHANGE?

The lesson of Liza and Henry is that it would be no more useful for me to try to tell you *how* to change than it would have been to tell you *whether* you should change. Rather, my job is to provide you with a structure for developing a plan and help you draw on your own strengths, skills, knowledge, and creativity to fill in that structure with pieces that feel like a good fit. Then, once you've begun to carry out your plan, I will guide you in evaluating its effectiveness and revising it accordingly.

The first principle for helping another person solve a problem is that the helper's job is not to solve the problem!

Why is it my role to act as a facilitator of your problem solving rather than an expert who supplies the answers? One reason was foreshadowed in the interplay between Henry and Liza—when authors (or other professionals) act like experts, those they're trying to help have little choice but to take on the role of passive recipients of expertise. Instead of empowering you to use your own resources, experts ask you to rely on theirs.

Now, admittedly, this can sometimes be just what a person with a problem wants: someone who can fix it. And when it comes to the kinds of problems that truly require specialist knowledge—repairing your car or your computer, prescribing medication for an illness, or surgically removing your appendix—this is usually a wise choice. But when it comes to changing behavior, situations, or personal patterns, *you* are the biggest expert on what will work for you and what will not. Of course, this does not mean that ideas or approaches from knowledgeable sources can't make a valuable contribution to the plan you formulate. But it does mean that formulating the plan is a job for the person who is going to put the plan into action and live with the consequences, not for a professional who cannot possibly be as invested in the outcome as you are.

Another important reason I will help you find your own answers rather than trying to supply them for you: You are more likely to carry out plans that you have developed than plans built out of advice given by others (including professionals). This is partly due to what is known as "the generation effect," the fact that people *remember* material they have produced better than material that is provided to them. But it is also due to the fact that a plan whose elements you have generated, pondered, and finally committed to is one that you will feel better *able* to carry out than one suggested to you by someone who does not know your unique combination of capacities and strengths.

And the final reason I won't try to answer the question of how you should make your change? There is no "answer." No matter what some experts may claim, the entire body of research on change shows that there is always more than one right way to do it. For many people who want to stop drinking, using drugs, or gambling, lose weight, or change their sexual behavior, Alcoholics Anonymous and its self-help/mutual support group cousins can be tremendously helpful. Yet it is equally true that many people who get sober or clean, give up gambling, change their eating patterns, or gain control over their sexual lives do so without any 12-step involvement at all. Medication for depression has brought millions of people relief—

> When it comes to succeeding at change, the question is not "What is the answer?" but "What is the right answer for me?"

yet so have a variety of psychotherapies in the absence of antidepressants. Some people find nicotine replacement (gum, patch, etc.) crucial in their efforts to quit smoking—yet most people who quit do so without these aids. And on and on it goes; there is no one-size-fits-all solution for any of the problems this book is intended to help you solve.

Your best chance of success will come from developing a plan that you're willing and able to carry out and that you feel confident will work for you if you put it into action. How well a plan or any of its components "fits" for you is as important to determine as whether there's evidence of its general effectiveness.

And just as there are many right ways to change, there is no foolproof form of help—and that very much includes this one. If any of the guidelines I share feels wrong to you or saps your motivation, trust yourself and disregard it! Nothing, including these guidelines, is right for everyone, and you will be the best judge of what works for you.

The good news? In my work I have helped people come up with an amazing variety of successful plans for change in a wide variety of problem areas. Some centered on elements that I'd seen other people use successfully, while others never would have occurred to me and yet turned out to be a perfect fit for the person who came up with it. There is every reason to believe that you, too, will be able to come up with a plan that's right for you.

WHAT WORKS?

I will describe the components of change plans as I help you develop yours in Chapter 7. But before we get there, it will be useful to keep in mind the general characteristics that distinguish approaches to change that work from ones that are less likely to accomplish what you want to accomplish.

Effective change plans are *specific*. Psychologist Peter Gollwitzer's research on "implementation intentions"[1] has shown that, when it comes to making relatively easy changes, it usually suffices just to decide what you want to do and then go ahead. But where more difficult changes are concerned, it's valuable to formulate a detailed plan for what you're going to do and how you're going to do it, as well as to prepare for bumps in the road so you're ready to handle them, and to make a firm commitment to sticking with the plan as best you can.

Effective change plans are *rewarding,* not all work and no play. Change can be hard, and there may be no way to avoid feeling at times like you're slogging along without much in the way of immediate results. To help you sustain the motivation that got you started and tolerate the difficult moments, it's important to build in opportunities to feel good about what you're doing and activities that provide pleasure and reduce stress.

Finally, effective change plans are *open to revision*, not carved in stone. No matter how thoughtful you are in developing a plan and how thorough it is, there's no way to know for sure how effective it will be (or rather, which parts will work as expected and which ones won't) until you've put it into practice. Good change plans resemble a jigsaw puzzle, with each piece in the right place and no extraneous pieces confusing the picture. For most people, it takes at least a couple of tries before they get it just right.

> The most important feature of a change plan is the readiness to change it.

THE WAY FORWARD

In the following chapters I will guide you in developing a change plan that fits your unique situation and problem-solving style, trying the plan out, evaluating how it's working, replacing the parts that don't quite fit with new ones that do, and trying it out again. In my experience, this will give you the best chance of succeeding at the changes you undertake. Let's get started.

---

[1]Stadler, G., Oettingen, G., & Gollwitzer, P. M. (2010). Intervention effects of information and self-regulation on eating fruits and vegetables over two years. *Health Psychology, 29,* 274–283.

7

Developing Your Plan

Effective plans for change include answers to these five questions[1]:

- What changes do I want to make?
- Why do I want to make these changes?
- What steps will I take to make these changes, and when will I take them?
- Whom can I call on for support in making these changes when I need it?
- What hurdles could arise as I'm making these changes, and what can I do to get past them?

To give you the best chance of success, I'm going to help you formulate your goals for change so you can stay aware of what you're working toward. I will help you describe your reasons for change so it's easy for you to remember why you're working hard to make these changes, especially when the going gets tough. I'll help you come up with steps that are concrete so you know what you're going to do to make the change and deal with different situations you encounter as you go about it. I'll also help you identify the people who are willing to support your efforts and the role each of them is willing to play, so when the time comes you know whom you can call on and what kind of support you can expect. And I will help you

---

[1]Miller, W. R., Zweben, A., DiClemente, C. C., & Rychtarik, R. G. (1992). *Motivational enhancement therapy manual* (Project MATCH Monograph Series, Vol. 2). Washington, DC: National Institute on Alcohol Abuse and Alcoholism.

anticipate as many potential hurdles as possible, so that you can be ready with ways of getting past them.

As you work through this chapter you'll complete a series of activities that prepare you to answer each of the five questions. Then you'll write your answers on a Personal Change Plan form, because having your entire plan in one place will make it easier to refer to it or revise whenever you like. As before, you can create your own change plan record in your journal or use the form available at *www.guilford.com/zuckoff-forms*.

GOALS FOR CHANGE

Goals are the intended endpoints of a process of striving; they are ahead of us and draw us on until they are achieved. During the last few activities you have most likely been identifying with increasing clarity the changes you want to make. The first step in change planning is to formulate *change goals* to guide you in identifying the steps you will need to take and monitoring your progress.

Change goals are concrete goals we can work toward that are achievable through our efforts. A goal of "being happy" is one that most of us would share. But to use that goal to drive an effective plan for change it would be important to begin by asking yourself, "How would my life have to change so that I would be happy?" Would having closer relationships be the key? Getting a job that satisfies and challenges me? Having enough money to live a particular lifestyle? Or if you had a goal of "good health," what would it take to get there? Losing weight? Exercising more? Improving your sleep? Reducing your stress?

Sometimes goals can be achievable but also a bit daunting, and people find themselves feeling overwhelmed rather than energized by the prospect of working toward them. This can happen when the goal is far off and it will take a lot of time to achieve; it can also happen when reaching the goal is complex and demanding.

For example, a person might have a goal of saving enough money to make an expensive purchase. Reaching that goal may not be complicated—but it's going to take some time to get there. A change plan to achieve a goal like this will need to include smaller milestones to confirm that progress is being made and reminders of why the long-term effort is worthwhile.

On the other hand, a student just entering college might have a goal of becoming a doctor. This goal is not only far off; it also requires the student to achieve a number of more immediate goals, each of which may require its own plan: how to get a good grade in organic chemistry; how to maintain a high grade point average for 4 years; how to complete a successful medical school application; how to get through the first year of med school; and so on. Breaking up complex, long-term goals into smaller and more manageable goals and focusing on achieving the goal that's closest while leaving work on the others until later can make the difference between a successful change process and one that gets derailed.

So with these guidelines in mind, please review and think about your responses to the most recent activities and identify your goals for change by asking yourself: "What changes do I want to make? How do I want my life to be different?" First, however, look at how your companions responded to these questions, shown below.

What Changes Do I Want to Make?

Alec

I want to get my life back in balance. To do that I think I need to do three things.

1. Make things better with Wendy—get us back on the same side.
2. Cut down on my drinking when I'm out with customers.
3. Carve out time to do things that I like doing—like getting back into shape and working on my car.

Barbara

1. Get to know my husband again and see what's possible for us.
2. Reenter the work force. Have a career!

Colin

1. Stop exploding at Paul. Find creative ways to change how I express anger.
2. Learn to communicate better with Paul about the things that upset me.

These goals are connected, but I think I need to work at both.

Dana

1. Go to graduate school to become a teacher!
2. Relate to my parents more like an adult—be honest with them about what I want to do.

Ellie

> 1. I might as well shoot high: get back to my prepregnancy weight. That's my main goal.
>
> 2. I want to get better at letting people help me when I need it.

As you read your companions' change goals you might have found yourself wondering how clear and achievable some of them are. Alec's goal of cutting down on his drinking might seem less concrete than it could be; perhaps it would be helpful for him to think about what a workable amount of drinking might be, although perhaps he'll reach that level of specificity when he begins to formulate his steps toward change. Ellie's goal of getting all the way back down to her prepregnancy weight seems very ambitious, especially in light of her struggles with confidence about change; perhaps she might be better off setting a more modest goal that she could feel more certain about achieving.

As you're thinking about *your* goals, ask yourself these questions:

- "Is this goal clear enough to be the basis for developing specific steps to achieve it?" If not, consider whether you can formulate it more concretely.

- "Does reaching this goal seem a long way off, or does it feel a bit overwhelming?" If the answer to either of these questions is "Yes," then consider whether there's a more limited, achievable version of the goal that you can start with.

Once you've written your responses in your change plan record in your journal or in the change plan form at *www.guilford.com/zuckoff-forms*, please read them aloud while listening to yourself before you go on to the next section, thinking about the changes you intend to achieve.

REASONS FOR CHANGE

The next step is to specify your reasons for making the changes you've listed. You've been doing a good deal of thinking and writing about what makes these changes important to you as you've completed the earlier activities. Now it's time to record your most important reasons in a way that is clear and easy to remember.

Life Goals

To help with this step I'd like to highlight a distinction between the change goals you just formulated—concrete goals that answer questions like "What do I need to accomplish to get where I want to go?" ("Cut down on my drinking" or "Get into graduate school") or "What kinds of changes would bring me closer to the way I want things to be?" ("Stop blowing up at my partner" or "Explore a new relationship with my husband")—and your *life goals*. Why is working toward change worth the effort? Because it serves your life goals, those global, organizing goals that provide your life with direction, meaning, purpose, and satisfaction. Life goals, which reflect your core values (although perhaps in ways you haven't quite made explicit), are the answers to questions like:

- "What do I want my life to be like?"
- "What do I most want to achieve or create for myself?"
- "When I picture the life I aspire to, how does it look?"

So to help you capture your most important reasons for change, I invite you first to identify and describe the life goals that achieving your change goals will bring you closer to. First, to bring your core values to the forefront, please reread your responses to the activity in Chapter 6, "The Values That Matter Most to Me." Then, imagine that it is 5 years from now and your life is exactly the way you want it to be. Try to picture things as clearly and in as much detail as possible and ask yourself: "What is my life like, not just in relation to the change I want to make, but overall?" Please read your response aloud after you've written it, listening to yourself as you do.

Consider your companions' descriptions of their life goals, shown below, before you write down your own in your journal or using the form at *www.guilford.com/zuckoff-forms*.

- -

What Do I Want My Life to Be Like?

Alec

I see the facts of my life in 5 years very much the way they are now—it's the quality that's different. I have just about everything I want, but I'm not enjoying it the way I could. I see more fun—with Wendy and Jen (well, she'll be 16, so I think I'd better have some of those fun times with her sooner), and our friends. Wendy and I talking and joking the way we used to. I see myself in my Camaro, which is looking great with the top down. I'm looking good, too—in top shape. And I still see myself working hard, doing what I need to do to make the sale, maybe with more supervisory responsibility, but without it taking over my life.

Barbara

Even though I'm not sure what I will be doing, I can imagine the feeling I will have doing challenging and fulfilling work, having a circle of stimulating colleagues, including a few who are my new friends. If I really let myself dream, I have discovered a new life with Steve, and we've fallen in love with each other again. I imagine us looking forward to seeing each other at the end of a day, being more intimate, challenging each other. And who knows? Maybe by then there will be grandkids!

Colin

This is what I picture: Paul and I are married. We're happier than we have ever been together. He has gained a deeper understanding of me, and I feel more accepted and contented. He feels safe with me and doesn't worry about my temper anymore. I'm still at my job, but I also have more time to devote to my own art since we're not wasting time and energy fighting. Maybe I have a studio and show my work in a gallery. Paul and I travel together; at least we will have gone to Greece, which we have both always wanted. Maybe for our honeymoon.

Dana

I picture myself in my first teaching job after completing my master's and student teaching. I could do that in 5 years. I'm still excited about what I'm doing. Every day I come home tired, but I spend lots of time preparing lessons and figuring out how to keep my students excited about learning. I have a whole new group of friends that I met in graduate school, but I still have my old friends, too. My family will be proud of me, and I will be pretty proud of myself. There will be so many areas of education that I'll be researching and exploring that I will have never-ending growth. I'll have my whole future ahead of me!

Ellie

I want my life to be fuller in many ways. In 5 years? I'm still thinner and more energetic and healthy and feeling good about myself. Gil and I are closer than ever, and the kids are all doing well. Maybe I'm not doing quite as much work at family gatherings—maybe I'm letting someone else take the lead for a change! But I'm doing more social things, going out more, laughing more. I imagine being lighter (in both senses of the word!). I want to feel more appreciative of the life that God has given me.

Why Change?

Now that you've reflected on your ultimate goals in addition to the thinking you've been doing about the changes you want to make, please ask yourself: "What are the most important reasons for me to make these changes?"

Again, first consider your companions' reasons for change, which appear below. Then write down your own reasons in your change plan record in your journal or using the change plan form at *www.guilford.com/zuckoff-forms* and read your response aloud while listening to yourself and thinking about the reasons you've identified.

Why Do I Want to Make These Changes?

Alec

I want to make these changes because I am not getting everything out of my life that I can, and I want more. I deserve to enjoy what I have worked very hard for, and I want to feel good and strong and loved and successful. Wendy deserves more, too, and Jen also. They deserve to have the husband and father I'm capable of being. I don't want to be the guy they're talking about when they say, "No one ever said on his deathbed, 'I wish I'd spent more time at work.'"

Barbara

Because I have to live with passion and I want to go on sharing my life with Steve. I have so much to give to life and to others and so much potential to grow and learn and love. It can't be contained, so I have to risk the safety and comfort I have for something more challenging and exciting and valuable.

Colin

I found something that not everyone gets in life: a soul mate. I want to take care of that gift, nurture it so that both of us can feel the way we want to feel with each other. I know I can do that now, because I am a creative and loving person and this is really what it would mean to be true to myself.

Dana

> The most important reason is that this is what I have to do to fulfill my higher purpose, which must guide and carry me through my life. Teaching is my calling, and it is the best thing I can do for myself and for the world. And once my family sees what this means to me and what I'm capable of, I know it will be what they want for me, too.

Ellie

> Life is not forever, and if I give up on myself now, I will not keep getting more chances. Doing this will make me happier, and Gil, too. And I think it's also what God wants for me.

- -

STEPS TOWARD CHANGE

The steps you will take to accomplish your change goals comprise the heart of the change plan. In general, the strategies that are most likely to lead to successful change are those that feel *challenging but doable*.

As we've seen before, experiences of success or failure have the strongest impact on our confidence for change. Choosing actions that have a high likelihood of success initially can lay a foundation of confidence for what may be harder steps to follow. At the same time, actions that feel a bit more challenging will give you a greater sense of satisfaction when you complete them, and mastering a challenge is a powerful way to strengthen your self-efficacy.

What if you're not sure how to gauge the difficulty level that's right for you? The answer depends on how you typically respond when you try something for the first time and it doesn't go the way you'd hoped. For some people, that's a signal to redouble their effort and refuse to take no for an answer. If that's you, then go ahead and take on a little more than you're sure you can manage. On the other hand, if you're more likely to feel discouraged and lose momentum, or if your confidence starting out isn't robust, then think about a smaller step if you're not sure how "doable" the one you're considering is. It's important to avoid overloading yourself when you're taking your first steps, and if you realize that something was easier to do than you expected, you can always increase the challenge you're taking on.

If at first you don't succeed . . . are you motivated or deflated?

Because people vary considerably in how much help they need or want in developing this part of their plan, I've organized this section as a sequence of activities. Whenever you feel confident that the actions you've identified will be all it takes for you to succeed at change, skip to the end of this section and complete the "Steps I Will Take" part of your change plan. Of course, you might realize that you feel sure about how you're going to achieve one goal you've formulated but feel less certain how to tackle another; in that case, you might choose to complete the activities later in the sequence only for the one you're uncertain about.

What Have You Already Thought Of?

The place to begin is with the thinking you've already done. By now you may have been trying on different strategies in your mind or even experimenting with change. So for each of your change goals, please ask yourself, "What steps have I already been thinking about taking?"

Consider the steps your companions have been thinking about, shown below, before you write down yours in your journal or in the form at *www. guilford.com/zuckoff-forms*.

- -

What Have I Already Been Thinking about Doing?

Alec

> 1. Come home a little earlier during the week. One night this past week, there was not a major reason to stay out longer, so I did go home. In the past I may have lingered anyway, but I felt like leaving, so I did. I could tell that Wendy was surprised and happy about it.
>
> 2. Not having that last drink or two. Stopping once everyone's loose and relaxed.
>
> 3. I've thought about checking out this new gym that's nearby. I have a membership to a gym that I don't like and never use. This one costs more, but it might be worth it.

Barbara

> 1. I've thought about different ways to spend more time with my husband, maybe find a new hobby or activity we can share.
>
> 2. I've been thinking about what kind of career I might want. I think it's too late for me to go back and finish law school. I did talk with a friend who started graduate school after her kids were grown, and I felt encouraged that she was able to do it. I've gone online a few times, looking at

> continuing education programs at different schools, but I haven't found anything that really grabbed me.

Colin

> I've been thinking that I need to get better at recognizing when I'm upset about something and exploring how to put it into words or even just make myself feel a little less upset before the feeling gets intense. It's a different approach. Also getting more interested in myself and expanding my options for feeling good. It sounds selfish, but it seems to be helping already. I've noticed that I feel more patient around Paul and better able to listen to him. But he hasn't made me mad yet, so I don't know whether this is enough.

Dana

> I know what I'm going to do. It feels like I've known all along and I just had to decide to do it.
>
> 1. I've been thinking about which schools to apply to and have already been narrowing down my options based on cost, location, and quality. I've looked at the schedule for the GREs, and I probably need to buy a practice exam book and start preparing. I want to contact the deans of the schools that look promising to talk to them about my interests and how well their programs match them. Also, about how feasible it would be for me to keep working part-time. I need to find out about financial aid, especially student loans—I've saved some money, but I might want to keep a safety buffer.
> 2. I've been mentally rehearsing where and how I'm going to talk with my parents.

Ellie

> 1. I honestly don't know where to start in thinking about the weight loss. Do I look at diets again? Find an exercise program? Talk with my doctor?
> 2. I have noticed myself not accepting help and have thought about what might happen if I would, or even asked people to help me. I've been trying to convince myself it would be okay.

What Strategies Have You Tried Before?

If you have tried before to make the change you're working on now, your own past experience can be an excellent resource for your current planning. (If you have never tried to make this change before, then please skip this activity and go on to the next one.)

Are you wondering, "How can past failures help me succeed?" Well, the question to ask yourself is "What do I mean by 'failures'?" When people try to change a behavior, situation, or pattern and end up less than 100% successful, many times they reduce the entire experience to a "failure" and write it off, even though they may have experienced partial success and there may be much to learn from the experience. For example, a person who has "failed" to quit smoking on multiple occasions may in fact have quit for days, weeks, or even months before resuming tobacco use. While the final outcome was disappointing, managing not to smoke for a period of time after smoking every day for years is no small accomplishment, and recalling what helped to make that happen can provide important clues about what might help again.

At the same time, the fact that the change could not be sustained also provides important information. In many cases, the problem was not that the strategies the person was using were useless or ineffective; rather, they may not have been enough by themselves. If so, developing a better plan might not mean throwing away everything you tried before; it might mean identifying the "missing pieces of the puzzle" and *adding* to the plan to fill in those gaps.

With this in mind, please think back to a time when you tried to make the change you're working on now and ask yourself: "What helped me make the progress I was able to make?" "What was I missing then that would have helped me go further?"

But first consider the recollections of your companions who have previously tried to change the same behavior, situation, or pattern they are planning to change now—shown below. Then write your answers in your journal or in the form at *www.guilford.com/zuckoff-forms*.

. . . .

Learning from Past Efforts to Make These Changes

Barbara

> This is the first time I've faced this kind of dilemma. I've never struggled this way before.

What helped me make the progress I was able to make?

> I wasn't making any progress.

What was I missing then that would have helped me go further?

> I've learned that not feeling I could talk with close friends about how I was feeling and feeling inhibited about being honest with my sister held me back from coming to terms with what I was struggling with.

Colin

> I was trying to control my anger with Paul for a while without much success.

What helped me make the progress I was able to make?

> I did do a little better with some of those anger management strategies—deep breaths, walking away. Like you said, I guess they weren't useless; they just weren't enough.

What was I missing then that would have helped me go further?

> What was missing was me really wanting to change the way I express anger. I was "halfhearted." You can't really get anywhere that way.

Ellie

> I have tried so many diets and programs. One time, after my first child was born, I went with a group of girlfriends to one of those programs for women to lose weight.

What helped me make the progress I was able to make?

> I did well for a while—better than my friends. I think being with a group was helpful. It was fun getting together with them, and I didn't feel so alone with my weight problem. I think it also helped to have some structure.

What was I missing then that would have helped me go further?

> When I got pregnant again, it kind of went out the window. I couldn't stay on the same diet, and then I never went back to it. By then, my friends dropped out because they weren't doing so well, and I didn't feel like doing it by myself. It got hard to make it to the meetings, too, time-wise.

- -

What Can Your Successes and Strengths Teach You?

The other way you can benefit from your experience is to think about the *successes* you've had when faced with challenging situations and the positive qualities or *strengths* you possess that have helped you cope with difficult situations in the past. You've already done this, of course, in the activity "A Difficult Challenge I Overcame" in Chapter 5 and the activities "The Positive Qualities That Are Most Characteristic of Me" and "When Two of My Positive Qualities Showed Themselves" in Chapter 3. Please go back and reread your responses to those activities now, and building on what you've already written, ask yourself "How can my successes and strengths help me with the changes I want to make now?"

Before you enter your own answers in your journal or in the form at *www.guilford.com/zuckoff-forms* consider your companions' answers, which appear below.

How Can My Successes and Strengths Help Me with the Changes I Want to Make?

Alec

No doubt it's going to take some discipline to reconfigure my life a bit. Like I'm going to have to think more about scheduling things like time to myself instead of just hoping it happens. I know I'm going to have to call on some of that patience I learned and not expect immediate results with Wendy. I'll have to give her time to catch on that I'm doing some things differently. Getting back in shape will take some patience and discipline, too.

Barbara

Reviewing those responses reminds me that I do very well with people. I can rely on my social skills and flexibility with others, particularly as I'm thinking about a new career. And my drive as well. As far as my marriage goes, I'm feeling different inside now, maybe more confident as a woman again, not just a wife and mother. It's exciting because, yes, I want to get to know Steve in new ways, but I think he'd also like getting to know me in new ways.

Colin

I've been focusing on how my creativity can help me step out of a situation where I feel stuck and explore alternatives. It's good to remind myself about how loving I can be and how much that means to Paul. That's the side of me I have to work on showing him more.

Ellie

When I'm doing something for other people out of love, or even when everyone is benefiting, I do pretty well, but if I'm doing it completely for myself, or people are focused on me, I get uncomfortable. I know that if I lose weight it would be good for my family, too, but not for some time, so I worry about being a burden getting there. The only way I'm going to be able to deal with this is by letting Gil in more.

Brainstorming

Brainstorming is a process for coming up with fresh ideas that might not occur to us otherwise. It's done in two phases, each of which utilizes a different type of thinking: *divergent* and *convergent*.

Divergent thinking is the kind of thinking you do when you're being creative—instead of looking for a single answer to a question or a solution to a problem, you generate a variety of options by allowing your mind to wander freely, looking at things from different angles and exploring as many ideas as you can think of without placing restrictions or judgments on the ideas you come up with. If your immediate reaction was "But I'm not creative," think again. Sure, artists, musicians, and others typically thought of as "creative types" think divergently all the time—trying out different words to see how the lyric they're writing sounds, or painting, looking, repainting, and then painting again. But so do salespeople who try out different versions of their "pitch," teachers who add and subtract components of their lesson plans and notice how this affects their students' learning, and parents who come up with new ways of presenting healthy foods to their growing children. The key to divergent thinking is giving yourself the freedom to be "wrong"—letting yourself play with different possibilities without worrying which one is the "right" one. Giving yourself permission to put off deciding which ideas you feel comfortable with and which ones could actually work will allow you to come up with new thoughts and make unexpected connections.

Then, once you've got a variety of possibilities, it's time for the second phase, a shift into convergent thinking—the kind you did when you took multiple-choice tests in school and tried to narrow the options down to the correct answer. This kind of thinking involves asking critical questions about the feasibility, desirability, practicality, and likelihood of success of each option you've identified, so that you can select the ones that are best for you.

To get you started, here are some guidelines for the "divergent" phase of the brainstorming process.

1. Give yourself a moment to get comfortable and clear your mind. Then start writing down every idea you can possibly think of that might help you with the change you're planning for. Don't filter out anything, no matter how impractical or even impossible it may seem. Wishing for a magic wand to change everything? Write it down! Think of something that someone has to help with but you don't think they will? Include that, too!

2. Search your memory for ideas you've heard, read about, or seen other people try. Suggestions that people have made in the past that you ignored or dismissed? Write those down, too. (Just keep in mind that you're not committing to *doing* any of these things at this point in the process.)

3. Think about possible sources of information about the behavior, situation, or pattern you want to change or about other strategies for addressing it. Are there websites or books that you might want to consult as part of your plan? Is there anyone—whether a person with special expertise or someone whose judgment you trust—you might want to talk to for advice, information, or guidance?

4. Be dogged and persistent: when you think you've thought of everything, think more. Read the ideas you've already written down and see if you can approach them from a different angle. Keep going until you absolutely can't come up with anything else.

Before you do some brainstorming of your own, take a look at the ideas your companions came up with, shown below. Then use your journal or the form at *www.guilford.com/zuckoff-forms* to write down your ideas.

. . . .

Brainstorming

Alec

(1) Wendy will be waiting with a smile on her face at least twice a week when I come home, with a great dinner and a bottle of wine for us, and we'll have a great night alone! (2) We make plans with friends at least one weekend night to go to a game and hang out together afterward at a bar or one of our houses. (3) We take a family vacation every summer like we used to, where I can relax, watch all of the kids enjoying each other, and no one complains if I have to respond to an occasional work call. (4) I could get a personal trainer. (5) I plan real quality time with Jen, and then I don't have to feel guilty about that, plus I won't feel like I'm missing out. (6) Maybe we can both join that new gym, Jen and I, and work out together. Maybe Wendy would want to join, too. (7) I start nursing my drinks a little more slowly on work nights, spreading them out. (8) I go to the gym in the morning, maybe, which will give me incentive to get to bed at night sooner—that might help me feel better and be more efficient during my work day, too. (9) I talk with my buddy about how he was able to cut out drinking altogether, even though I'm not planning to go that far, just to see if he has any good tips. (10) I was thinking about how easy it would be if there was a gym at the office, with a shower—that would save a lot of time. (11) I wonder if some clients might be

more interested in having lunch meetings, rather than doing business at a bar. (12) I'd love to find a group of guys who work on cars. (13) A while back, Wendy and Jen were asking if we could put an addition on the house with an indoor pool and a party area so that we could do more entertaining. (14) Talk with guys who took early retirement, like my brother-in-law, to see if I could afford it, then open my own business. (15) Clean out the basement, get it finished, and turn one corner of it into a mini gym with a huge plasma TV. (16) Add a pool table to the other side and a mini bar and finally finish that game room like we've been talking about for years.

Barbara

1. Taking a long weekend away with Steve at one of those relationship resort places, to rejuvenate our marriage. A trip to Israel. Steve and I take ballroom dancing lessons. We go to a nude resort together somewhere in Europe. Learning a sport together or trying something that he has always wanted to try, like taking exotic cooking classes together or wine tasting. Attending theater or lectures with him.

2. Meeting with women who have started their careers later in life. Attending lectures in different areas to see if any of them excite me. Going to a spa or a meditation retreat to get more in touch with me. What if it's not too late to finish law school? I could visit my old law school and see if any of the professors I liked are still teaching there. I could take one to lunch. Get a new hairstyle. Buy some new clothes that are more professional, not part of my Mom image. Maybe find a life coach.

Talking with my friends and sister will definitely help with both.

Colin

I have this fantasy of us coming together and baring our souls to each other—everything, our deepest insecurities, frustrations, desires, and so forth, like in the encounter groups of the sixties. Someone told me to get a punching bag to work out my anger when I'm mad. I read somewhere that couples in conflict should take tae kwon do together—supposedly it would give me more of that good type of self-control, and it might make Paul more able to understand me. I was thinking about couple therapy, to get to know each other more deeply, not fix my "anger problem." Collecting quotes, images, songs, and poems that capture my feelings and putting them all around me, like those Post-Its I used to learn French, to remind me to pay more attention to how I'm feeling, especially when I'm upset. Working on my own art is so important, so I'm picturing that new studio space. Practice putting my deeper emotions into words, rather than only in my artwork. Learning about Paul's inner world, the hurt especially, and doing a painting or even designing part of our home around it, as a reminder and a new start. Volunteering to do artwork for a local shelter for abuse victims. Taking yoga. Getting a weekly massage. Being open with our closest friends about these new changes. Asking Paul more directly for the sort of understanding and acceptance that matters to me. Just being more open in general with him. Take meditation classes. Go into analysis. Run across the country like Forrest Gump!

Ellie

Talk to Gil about what I want to do. Ask him for support. Let the whole family know that I need help to try to do this once and for all. Change the foods we keep in the kitchen. Go away to a "fat camp" for a month! See if a group of friends want to do this with me. (This is making me nervous.) Get that stomach-stapling operation. Go to church every day. Pray more. Join a water aerobics class for women. Join Weight Watchers online. Do one of those programs that delivers meals to your house. Go to Overeaters Anonymous. Enter the <u>Biggest Loser</u> competition on TV! Get my jaw wired shut! Take diet pills. Become a vegetarian like my daughter.

Here's one more prompt to help you draw every drop of water from the well. Imagine again that it's 5 years from now and your life is exactly how you'd hope it would be. Now ask yourself these questions: "How did I get here? What did I have to accomplish? What steps did I take, and why did they work?"

Consider your companions' responses, shown below, before answering for yourself and recording your thoughts in your journal or in the form at *www.guilford.com/zuckoff-forms.*

Looking Back from an Ideal Future

Alec

What I had to do was to keep Wendy, Jen, and myself happy. I did that by finally setting firm limits on how I spent my time. I planned times with my family each week so they wouldn't get pushed aside, but I still kept on top of work and even got that promotion. Part of what I learned was that taking better care of myself physically made me more efficient at work. So I cut back on drinking and worked on my body. I spent more alone time with Wendy, so we both felt we were getting what we needed. At first I had to be patient, because she had some leftover resentment about the times we were more disconnected. I hung in there and made sure each week we were having relaxed, fun times. And I spent more quality time with Jen and discovered that she didn't need more than that from me. But those quality hours were very important and I protected them, so she knew how much she mattered to me.

Barbara

I went back to my former college and looked into their graduate programs. I spoke with women who were successful later in life, and I discovered that I could do it, too. And I did. I went back to law school. And here I am with a growing career. When I had doubts, I talked to other women, and they shared their struggles with me, and that kept me encouraged and going forward. And I have a really strong marriage now. I got the courage up to tell Steve how I was feeling. He had no idea, and at first he was overwhelmed. I had to slow down and listen a lot. We took some risks with each other and spent time alone together and found that our relationship could grow and thrive. I had some doubts about this too, but I had my friends and my sister to support me.

Colin

It took a lot of steps to get here, mostly involving my willingness to look deeply into myself and make changes, sharing myself more fully and deeply with Paul, and learning a lot more about him and appreciating and loving him. The steps I took were much more indirect than direct. While I worked on learning to express my anger differently and in a better way, the other changes that we both made resulted in my being less angry overall and caring more about making things better in our environment and safer for Paul. The safer he felt, the more I understood him and felt safer with him, and the more I could open up and share more of my feelings with him, and then he felt even safer and made me feel more accepted. It just seemed to grow reciprocally. But I did put effort into paying more attention to myself when I got upset and making sure that what mattered to me most got expressed, but not in a hostile way. I took time when I got angry, instead of reacting, and I thought through what mattered to me in those moments. That helped me see that the ways I was getting angry before weren't helping me any more than they were helping Paul or our relationship.

Ellie

It wasn't easy. I asked everyone in my life to help me, I worked really hard at a good diet, and I added exercise, some of it in fun ways. I had a group of friends who were losing weight with me at the same time, and they were really nice, and we supported each other. I had to tell people, especially Gil, when I felt discouraged and when I cheated or wanted to give up. It was really hard to do that. And I prayed a lot and asked God for help.

Now that you have a collection of brainstormed ideas at your disposal it's time for the "convergent" phase of the process: evaluating your options and deciding which to include in your change plan. Questions to ask yourself as you're doing the evaluations include:

- "How likely is this step to work?"
- "How practical will it be for me to put it into action?"
- "Is there any downside to doing this? If so, does the potential upside outweigh it?"
- "How well does it fit with my way of dealing with life and moving through the world?" (The best components of a change plan are those that feel like a good fit for you.)

As you read what you've written, don't be too quick to dismiss ideas that might seem a little "out there" or unconventional if they also hold some appeal. One of the lessons I've learned in helping people develop change plans for different problems is that solutions some might view as wrongheaded and likely to fail or just not serious enough can work perfectly well for the person who thought of them. Since none of the steps you're including will be written in stone, the worst that will happen is that you'll discover the idea wasn't workable after all and discard it. On the other hand, you might be surprised at what a good fit some of those ideas can turn out to be.

Some years ago a young woman talked with me about wanting to get into better physical shape but hating exercise. She explained how self-conscious she felt at health clubs and exercise classes and how boring she found it to go running and what a terrible athlete she was. I asked her what she *did* like to do, and she mentioned that she loved to dance. When I asked her what she loved about it, she talked excitedly about feeling the music, moving to the rhythm, losing herself in it . . . Before I could say anything more, she looked at me with a gleam in her eye: "I could dance, couldn't I? In my room, alone, where I won't care what I look like. It doesn't have to be 'exercise.'" Months later, she contacted me to say she was still dancing and feeling great.

The Steps I Will Take

Please describe the steps you will take to accomplish each of your goals for change. Organize them by listing each of your goals, followed by their respective steps. Be sure to decide *when* you are going to take each of the steps and include that as well. Before you formulate your own steps for each change goal, review the steps your companions have decided to take, shown below. Then record your thoughts in your change plan record in your journal or in the change plan form at *www.guilford.com/zuckoff-forms*.

What Steps Will I Take to Make These Changes?

Alec

To get my life back in balance I will do these three things:

Make things better with Wendy—get back on the same side.

1. I'm going to plan ahead to be home earlier most work nights, starting this week.

2. I am going to tell Wendy this week that I want to have at least one night a week that is reserved for spending time alone together and one night a week that we make a plan with friends.

3. The first night we spend together I'm going to talk to her about respecting each other. I'm going to tell her that I realized that it wasn't respectful of me to brush off her feelings about my drinking and coming home late and that I felt she could have been more respectful toward me in talking to me about it.

Cut down on my drinking when I'm out with customers.

1. This week I'm going to start nursing my drinks when I'm out with customers and cutting out at least the last one of the night.

2. I'm going to talk with Jim at work about what kinds of things he did to stop drinking. Not sure how soon I can do this, but I'll see if he wants to have coffee.

Carve out time to do things that I like—like getting back into shape and working on my car.

1. I am going to check out the new gym in our area next weekend. I'm also going to talk with Wendy and Jen about possibly joining with me, and I'm going to tell them why.

2. I think I will hold off on the car until later—this seems like enough for now.

Barbara

Get to know my husband again and see what's possible for us.

1. I will talk with Steve about spending more quality time together. I'm going to tell him that I miss our closeness and feel like it's been a long

time since we've had time together. I don't think he'll feel threatened by that. I want it to sound like an invitation he'll welcome. I will do this next weekend.

2. If he responds well, I will tell him I'd like to go out to dinner the weekend after that. At that dinner I'll feel him out about doing something new together, as a first step.

3. If that goes well, I will have the big conversation with him, telling him how I've been feeling and how much more I want to share with him. I can't say exactly when I'll feel ready to do that.

Reenter the work force. Have a career!

1. I will look into what it would take for me to finish law school. This week.

2. I will find women who have restarted careers at my age and ask them about the challenges and if they're glad they did it. This might take a couple of weeks.

3. I will tell Steve my plan to visit our law school and see what he thinks about it. I am fairly sure that he'll encourage me, especially if he sees my excitement and trepidation.

4. I am going to talk with my sister, friends, and family about what I find out from my visit.

Colin

Stop exploding at Paul. Find creative ways to change how I express anger.

Learn to communicate better with Paul about the things that upset me.

1. Starting now, I'm going to work on being less reactive by using deep breaths, and if I can't calm myself I'm going to walk away instead of exploding.

2. Starting now, I'm going to collect quotes, images, songs, and poems and put them around me to remind me to pay more attention to how I'm feeling, especially when I'm upset.

3. I'm going to look into classes on meditation, because I need more skills to soothe myself.

4. I am going to spend more time on my own art. I'll start by telling Paul I want to take a few hours every weekend just to work on my own projects.

5. I'm going to start looking into studio space. I'm not sure whether I want to create it in our home or I could rent a small space somewhere, so I need to explore that.

6. I'm going to practice expressing all my feelings in words. I'm not sure whether I'll need help with that. I might think about finding a therapist.

7. I want to ask Paul to talk to me about the times when he felt the worst when I got angry at him. I'm going to wait a little while to do this because it will be hard for me not to get defensive and I don't want that.

8. I will make a painting of what I've learned about Paul once we start really talking.

Dana

Go to graduate school to become a teacher!

1. Contact the deans of the three schools where I'm thinking of applying, to talk to them about my interests and how well their programs match them. Also ask them about working part-time while I'm in their program. I'll send the e-mails today.

2. Contact the financial aid offices of those schools to find out what's available. This week. Also look online for information on student loan options.

3. Buy a practice exam book for the GRE this week and start preparing to take the test.

4. Complete applications for the schools I decide on!

5. Contact my college about getting transcripts sent where I apply. After applications.

Relate to my parents more like an adult—be honest with them about what I want to do.

1. Call my mom and say I want to take her and my dad out to dinner at our favorite restaurant because I want to discuss something with them. I will do this after I've collected all the information I need to be able to talk with them about what I'm doing.

2. Tell them about my decision at dinner. They might be surprised, and I might have to explain how I came to my decision and why it's right for me, but they might even expect it after hearing me talk about this so much. Either way, I'll be ready.

3. Talk about the financial aspects in ways that will be reassuring. Explain exactly how I'm going to manage it.

Ellie

Get back to my prepregnancy weight.
Get better at letting people help me when I need it.

1. My first step is to talk to Gil. Explain to him that I want to go about trying to lose weight a different way this time and that it means a lot to me and that I really need his support.

2. I think I will ask a few friends to help me along. I am going to put a flyer up at church for a women's support group for anyone who wants to lose weight, who is at least 20 pounds overweight (I don't want to be in with

> the skinny ones who think they're overweight but aren't!). I'll organize it, but we'll all lead it together. We'll help each other.
>
> 3. I am going to research places like Weight Watchers and others to see if I can find out which are the most effective diet programs.
>
> 4. I'm going to replace my comfort foods with healthy snacks.
>
> 5. I am going to pray about this more, starting right away. I am going to ask for God's help and guidance in talking with Gil and the others in my life.
>
> 6. I will make an appointment with my doctor, get a physical (I'm overdue), and ask what kind of exercise is safe for me to start doing. I'll call for an appointment this week, but he probably won't see me for a couple of weeks.

At this point the path toward change might seem very clear and you may feel confident in the strategies you've come up with. Don't worry, though, if you feel more like you've made a good start but still need to add more pieces to the puzzle, or even if you're doubtful that the ideas you've come up with will be effective enough. There are still two more components of the change plan to be completed, and those elements can make the difference between a plan that feels shaky and one that feels like a solid foundation for change.

SOURCES OF SUPPORT

The people in our lives can play an important positive role in supporting our steps toward our change goals. As we saw in Part I, however, they can also help keep us stuck, sometimes despite the best of intentions. My purpose in this section is to help you identify the kind of help that will actually feel like constructive support and decide who in your life may be willing and able to provide it.

One of the most powerful ways that people can support our efforts to change is by believing in our ability to achieve it. Research on *self-fulfilling prophecies* has repeatedly demonstrated that other people's positive expectations of our performance can influence our likelihood of success. These "Pygmalion effects" (so named by psychologist Robert Rosenthal after the Greek myth of an artist who fell in love with the sculpture of a beautiful woman he'd carved and in doing so brought the sculpture to life)[2] have

---

[2]Rosenthal, R., & Jacobson, L. (1968). *Pygmalion in the classroom*. New York: Holt, Rinehart & Winston.

been found between schoolchildren and their teachers, employees in large organizations and their managers, and people receiving professional counseling and their therapists. For example, when alcohol rehabilitation program counselors (and no one else) were told that clients entering treatment had taken a test that could determine their potential for recovery, and that certain clients had "high alcohol recovery potential (HARP)," not only did the counselors later rate those clients as more motivated for change, but those clients were much more successful in changing their alcohol use than other clients in those programs—even though the test was fake and the only difference between the HARP clients and all the others was that the counselors *believed* the HARP clients had greater potential to recover.[3]

How do other people's expectations of us influence our behavior? In at least two ways. People who expect us to succeed treat us differently, often without even realizing it; they give us more attention and are warmer and more nurturing, but they also ask more of us and give us more opportunities to live up to their expectations. They also convey a message of hope and faith in us that we, in turn, take to heart, increasing our belief in ourselves and our confidence that we can succeed.

Unfortunately, research also shows that the opposite can be true—when people we're close to expect us to fail, the way they treat us and the message we take from them can lead to decreasing confidence and a greater likelihood of failure. (These have been called "Golem effects," after the mythological monster whose evil derived from the negative expectations of those around it.) So when it comes to deciding whom to call on for support as you work toward change, it's important to select people you feel sure believe in you and will be willing to offer you the patience, care, and assistance you'll be looking for from them.

The other important thing to think about as you're deciding whom to call on for support is the *kind* of support you'd like to have. People differ greatly in what they find helpful. Some do best when they have someone they can talk to about what they're doing and any struggles they're having, knowing that their support person will just listen without judgment or offer encouragement. Others want much more active supports: people who will offer advice, point out things they've missed, or otherwise give them guidance. Still others don't want to talk at all about the changes they're making; all they want is someone who, if asked for a favor or some practical assistance, will be there without having to go into a long discussion of why the help is needed.

---

[3]Leake, G. J., & King, A. S. (1977). Effect of counselor expectations on alcoholic recovery. *Alcohol Health and Research World, 11,* 16–22.

As with every other aspect of your change plan, there is no "right" way to use others' support. What matters is that you're clear in your own mind about what sort of support will be helpful for you and who you can get it from.

With this guidance in mind, please think now about the people in your life and ask yourself: "Whom can I call on for support?" and "How can they support me?" If you're not certain at first, a helpful approach to thinking about this is to return to your picture of how you would like your life to be 5 years from now and ask yourself: "Who helped me? How did they help?"

Before you record the supports you've identified in your change plan record in your journal or in the change plan form at *www.guilford.com/zuckoff-forms*, consider the supports your companions came up with, which appear below.

. . . .

Supports for Change

Alec

Whom can I call on for support?	How can they support me?
Wendy?	I'm not a big "support" guy. It would help if Wendy recognizes that I'm trying and shows some patience, like understanding if there are still some nights I need to come home late.
Jen?	I don't want to lean on Jen—it's more that I want to be there for her.
My buddy Jim at work	Jim, though—he's a good guy, and I respect him. Maybe it would be good to hear more about what he went through and what it's been like for him to make such a big change.

Barbara

Whom can I call on for support?	How can they support me?
My sister, for sure	Having my sister as my confidante and cheerleader again would feel great. Once I share what I've decided with her I think our relationship will get back to normal, which will be a relief.

| Maybe a couple of close friends | One of my friends in particular will understand how it feels to try to restart a career at this age—I know she'll build up my confidence, and she'll probably have some good practical advice also. |
| And, I hope, Steve. | I know Steve will support my decision to go back to work, and I'll have whatever financial resources I need. I hope he'll be able to share my eagerness to reconnect. |

Colin

Whom can I call on for support?	How can they support me?
Paul, of course	By being patient and understanding, particularly if I slip up.
Maybe a therapist	If I find a therapist, I'd want him to be a good listener but also someone who can pick up on mistakes I'm making and help me rethink what I'm doing.
Two of our closest friends, Judy and Dan	Actually, that's something that Judy is really good at. I wonder if I could talk to her about all these things I'm thinking and see if she thinks I'm on the right track—kind of a reality check.

Dana

Whom can I call on for support?	How can they support me?
My family	It would be awesome if my parents tell me that they believe in me and think this is a good direction for me.
My friends	I know my friends will be excited for me when I tell them what I'm doing—some of them have been telling me I was selling myself short—I can't wait to see their faces.
My spiritual community	My spiritual community is a place where I can get rejuvenated and feel at peace. I've kind of drifted away from them lately—it's time for me to get back with them.

Ellie

Whom can I call on for support?	How can they support me?
Gil	The best way Gil could support me is to be the way he was when he helped me get on that plane. He made me feel like I could do it and like I was never alone. I hope he can be that way about this.
Maybe my kids too	If my kids would accept having less junk food in the house, especially my comfort foods, it would help a lot. Gil, too.
My extended family	I could talk to my sister and ask her not to say things like "Go ahead, try some; just a little won't hurt."

HURDLES AND HOW YOU'LL GET PAST THEM

Your final step before putting your plan into action is to anticipate the challenges that could arise as you carry it out and prepare for how to cope with them.

Why prepare for problems instead of just hoping that all will go smoothly? The simple answer is: Better safe than sorry. But the more thorough answer is that it's much easier to handle new challenges if you've already put some thought into what you can do about them.

By definition, taking steps toward change takes you out of your comfort zone and puts you into unfamiliar territory. Under those conditions, you can't rely as you usually would on your "instincts"—which are really the responses you've made repeatedly in similar situations that have become "second nature" to you. In fact, it's likely that your instincts will tell you to act *in the very ways you're trying to change* because that's what you've done so many times before. This is why, for example, people who are working hard not to smoke (or drink or avoid conflict instead of acting assertively) and have been having some success, but start to feel the strain of working at change, will find themselves thinking, "I need a break, so maybe if just this once I have a cigarette/drink a beer/let another person override my wishes. . . ."

> It's easier to cope with the unexpected if you're already expecting it.

If you're forced to decide on the spot how to respond to an unexpected hurdle, you'll be trying to problem-solve while coping with the handicaps of stress and other demands on your attention. It's not likely that you'll do your best thinking under those conditions. You might come up with something that's just workable or not even workable or maybe nothing at all—and the pull of the behavior that is most familiar (and thus easiest to do) will be too great to resist successfully.

So please review the steps you're planning to take and ask yourself: "What could make it challenging to take those steps? What could make it hard for me to carry them out? What might get in the way of sticking with the plan I've made?" And once you've identified all the potential challenges you can think of, ask yourself: "What could I do to overcome these challenges?"

Consider the hurdles your companions identified and how they planned to overcome them, shown in the table below, before recording your own in your change plan record in your journal or in the change plan form at *www.guilford.com/zuckoff-forms*.

. . . .

Hurdles and Solutions

Alec

What hurdles could arise?	What will I do to overcome them?
1. I could get a client who's big on everyone ordering round after round and notices if you don't keep up.	1. The bartender where we take clients has known me for years—I could ask him to water down my drinks. That doesn't solve the time problem, though. If I explain to Wendy what I'm doing, I think she'd accept that I can't always get home as early as I want.
2. I could discover that I'm not able to work out like I used to, or my doctor could tell me that I'm not in good enough shape to do heavy workouts.	2. I could start slow. Or maybe switch to swimming for a while first.
3. I could be too tired a bunch of days in a row and skip the gym. If that happens, I might be tempted to give up.	3. I think Jen would get a kick out of it if I asked her to be my workout monitor and encourager, even if she doesn't want to go work out with me.

Barbara

What hurdles could arise?	What will I do to overcome them?
1. Steve might not respond to my approach to reconnecting with him the way I hope.	1. Not panic or give up. Remind myself that it's been a long time since we were intimate in every sense and that he hasn't been thinking about this the way I have, so this could really confuse or hurt him at first. That will help me be patient and understanding and give him time to come around. If he still doesn't respond, ask him to go to marriage counseling. And if he doesn't want what I want, finally, I will have to think about how to end our marriage in a way that allows us to go on being partners in loving our children. This is very sad to think about, but not as scary anymore.
2. I could discover that even though he's willing to try, the sparks don't fly for me.	2. Look into guidance for rejuvenating your sex life later in marriage. If we didn't make headway, think about sex therapy? I'm not sure he would be open to that. Ultimately, it's the same as #1.
3. Going back to law school could turn out to be more than I can handle.	3. Back to the drawing board and keep looking for another direction. I'm not going to give up on myself.

Colin

What hurdles could arise?	What will I do to overcome them?
1. Deep breaths and walking away might not be enough to keep me from exploding.	1. Do more research to find other techniques I can use. Get to work fast on learning to meditate.
2. I might get angry so quickly that I'm yelling before I even realize it.	2. This is a hard one. The only thing I can think of is if Paul can accept

	that I will have setbacks even though I'm trying. Maybe if I talk to him about this up front he'll be able to help me.
3. It might be harder than I think to start telling Paul how I feel more often.	3. This would be a good thing to practice in therapy. Maybe I shouldn't just consider it but start looking for a therapist now.
4. Some of the resentments I felt toward Paul could come back.	4. This one scares me. Maybe it would help to keep rereading what I wrote when I had my insight about my feelings for Paul until this isn't a risk.

Dana

What hurdles could arise?	What will I do to overcome them?
1. I don't get into any programs I apply to.	1. Apply to more!
2. They don't offer me financial aid.	2. I could find a part-time or night program and work full-time.
3. My parents get mad when I tell them what I'm going to do.	3. I don't think they will. But if they do, I have to be ready to stay calm and hold firm. No yelling. Keep loving them.

Ellie

What hurdles could arise?	What will I do to overcome them?
1. Maybe no one will want to join my support group.	1. I guess I could try going to a weight loss group that's already organized.
2. I could get discouraged if my weight doesn't come down.	2. I would need Gil to really encourage me to keep going, even if I haven't made much progress and I'm miserable.
3. I could get invited to a mandatory work lunch and have really tempting food put in front of me.	3. I could eat only part of my meal or I could let myself enjoy the meal but go back to my regular diet afterward.

4. We could have family events or vacations or holidays that throw off my discipline.	4. I'd have to prepare before I go. Tell myself not to cheat. Maybe bring my own food.
5. I could feel tired or get sick or injure myself exercising or not be able to keep it up.	5. Just keep going. Not make excuses. Go back as soon as I can after I get better.

COMMITTING TO YOUR PLAN

If your planning has gone as intended, you now have a clear picture in mind of what your change goals are and how you're going to accomplish them. The final step is to decide whether you're confident in the plan you've made and ready to make a commitment to carrying it out. So please read all your responses on the change plan form out loud, listening to yourself as you do, and then ask yourself: "Is this what I am going to do?"

Here are your companions' responses to this question:

- *Alec:* "Definitely. It's going to make things better for everybody."
- *Barbara:* "I feel as though I've found me again. It's scary and exciting, and I feel alive. I know I'm on the right track."
- *Colin:* "Yes. I can't wait to talk to Paul about it."
- *Dana:* "I'm already doing it! It feels great."
- *Ellie:* "I don't know how confident I am, but I will try."

If you too answered "yes" to this question, then you will be putting your plan into action. A window of opportunity for change opens when people decide what they're going to do and make a commitment to do it. How long the window stays open can vary—but experience says those who step through that window once it opens are those who are most likely to capitalize on the momentum toward change that they've developed.

THE WAY FORWARD

You've come a long way from the ambivalence you started with in Chapter 1 to this place, on the brink of action. I hope, if you've worked your way through the activities between there and here, that you feel a sense of accomplishment already, because resolving ambivalence and committing to change is no small feat.

At the same time, in another sense, you are just beginning. And as you prepare to take that famous "first step" with which even a journey of a thousand miles proverbially begins, I want to remind you that, no matter how hard you worked on it, and how thoughtful and careful you were, the plan you've made will very likely not be your final plan.

It's possible that things will go smoothly and the only adjustments you have to make in your plan are minor ones. This, of course, is what I wish for all the people I've tried to help. But there is no way to anticipate all the possible obstacles that could arise as you carry out your plan; life may throw you a curve ball, or something might catch you off guard. You will learn things as you change, and new ideas about how to get where you're trying to go may come to you that you can't think of now, because you haven't yet learned what you need to know. On the other hand, you might discover that some of the steps you planned to take don't work as expected or that some of the supports you thought you could rely on are not so reliable. There's no way to know ahead of time which ones those will be—but don't be too surprised if something that seemed like a good idea at first turns out not to be such a good fit after all.

The important thing to keep in mind is that none of these things is a sign that you haven't done what you needed to do before you came to this point, or that you're not going to succeed at change. Quite the contrary: the experiences I've just described are part and parcel of the normal process of change for most people. And this is why the next chapter is devoted largely to helping you revise your original plan based on your experience in trying it out.

How soon you should continue on to Chapter 8 will depend in part on the time frames you've chosen for carrying out the steps you've formulated. For many people, working on their plan for two or three weeks gives them enough experience to begin to judge how effective the plan is and where it might need some revision. The activities of Chapter 8 will help you decide what sorts of changes to make to your plan so you can reach your goals.

So if you hit some bumps as you start to work on change, remember that the saying "the best laid plans of mice and men oft go awry" is a cliché because it is so true. Don't get discouraged or, worse, get down on yourself if some things don't go as planned. There are steps yet to take on your journey, and I (and your companions in change) will be accompanying you for some time longer.

8

Revisiting, Revising, and Regrouping

There's a line from Samuel Beckett's *Worstward Ho* that's long been a favorite of mine: "Ever tried. Ever failed. No matter. Try again. Fail again. Fail better." Now, Beckett is no one's idea of an optimist, and I'm hoping that you've already begun to see some success from the steps you've been taking. But the spirit of perseverance this line expresses—and the acceptance that struggles and stumbles are to be expected when you're trying to achieve something important—are common threads among successful changers.

The plan you developed can be thought of as a starting point in a process of learning about what you need to do and the resources you need to have to get where you want to go. That starting point might be robust enough to carry you along with little alteration—or it might require adjustments or even a change of direction. My focus now is on helping you reflect on your experience of putting your plan into action and use what you've learned so far to identify missing pieces and unhelpful elements.

REFLECTING ON YOUR PROGRESS

I will guide you through a detailed review of each aspect of your change plan later in this chapter. But before digging into the details it's helpful to take a step back and look at the big picture. How are you feeling about your progress overall?

It's natural, when actions don't go exactly as planned, to focus more on what has gone wrong than on what has gone right. In some ways this can be constructive—targeting problems can focus energy on how to solve them. But it can also undermine your morale when you most need to keep your spirits up. Worse, it can distract you from noticing how much has gone well and using that awareness to build on the success you've had.

So I'd like you to start by thinking about the positive progress you've made since you began working toward your goals. Please ask yourself: "What has gone well?" Before recording your success so far in your journal or in the form at *www.guilford.com/zuckoff-forms*, consider your companions' reflections shown below.

. . . .

What Has Gone Well So Far?

Alec

I feel pretty good about how many things I've done. I've been getting home earlier, and it hasn't been as tense between Wendy and me. I decided to try texting her to tell her when I was coming home, and I was surprised by how much she appreciated that. Interesting how little things make a difference. I've been feeling a little more energetic—maybe it's from spending less time out or not having that last drink. I'm not sure. I also checked out that new health club, and it looks pretty good. Things are moving along.

Barbara

I've been spending more time with Steve and testing the waters; I think I'll know when the time is right to take it further with him. We did get season tickets to the theater—he was surprised but very responsive when I asked him about that. I found out that if I want to get a law degree I'll have to reapply and start over—I should have anticipated that in light of how long it's been. But after browsing websites dedicated to adults who are considering resuming their education I'm even more confident that I can do it. I have a date to take a friend of a friend who got her degree after her kids were grown to lunch next week and an appointment with the dean of my old law school the week after that. Progress!

Colin

It's been up and down, to be honest. But I'm supposed to focus on just the good things here. The main one is that I have not blown up or had any fights with Paul. I've been able to walk away when I've been frustrated and resist the temptation to complain that I'm doing all the work, which I know is not true. I told him about my Post-It notes idea, and he seemed to think it was pretty cute. Instead of just quotes and songs to remind me to pay attention to my feelings, I'm also writing messages about what I appreciate about him, and that seems to be helping, too. We've had some nice evenings together, and he was supportive when I talked to him about working on my own art on the weekends. The frustration is mostly about feeling Paul keeping his distance from me emotionally. But I'm in this for the long haul, and it does help to remind myself that there are some good signs.

Dana

It's going just like I hoped. I have my study materials for the GRE and am almost through the applications. My schools are rank ordered, although I keep going back and forth on where I'll be happiest. The money might be the deciding factor, because financial aid for grad school is mostly about loans, but there are some programs that help you if you're going into teaching and it looks like I will be able to work part-time. I'm going to talk to my boss and see if it might even be an option where I am now. I'm ready to make that call to my parents and take the next big step.

Ellie

I'm sorry, but I can't say too much that's positive. I talked to Gil, and he tried to be helpful. But I haven't really done much of what I said I was going to do. It all sounded good when I was writing it, but then the whole thing felt too overwhelming. I honestly don't know what comes next. Maybe this really is impossible for me.

People can vary widely in their initial progress when working toward change. If, like Alec, Barbara, Colin, and Dana, you were able to describe at least some ways in which you are seeing progress toward your goals—even if everything is not going smoothly—please skip the next section and move ahead to revisiting and revising your change plan.

But if, like Ellie, your momentum has stalled, or it's hard to find anything positive in what you've done so far, please go on to the next section for a different approach.

REGROUPING THROUGH SELF-OBSERVATION

If you're reading this, there's a good chance that you're feeling pretty discouraged. You made a commitment to change and began working in good faith to implement your plan. Now you might be wondering whether there's still reason to believe in a better outcome or whether you should just give up and spare yourself further disappointment.

Rather than trying to keep on plowing ahead, all the while feeling hope and enthusiasm draining away, it's better to pause and regroup when our best-laid plans go awry. Fortunately, there is a reliable way to do just that.

Do you remember Donal, introduced in Chapter 5? He had managed on his own to stop using a variety of substances he'd depended on since he was a teenager—except for marijuana, which he was relying on more heavily than ever. He had sought help because, although he very much wanted to free himself from this last drug as well, he could not imagine getting through his days without some way of dampening the loneliness he'd always felt and the anger it triggered in him—and nothing he'd found so far could provide the immediate and lasting relief that marijuana brought.

In our first meeting, Donal told me with considerable apprehension (after describing his dilemma) that he knew he had to "bite the bullet" and somehow get himself to quit smoking weed. I invited Donal to talk about *why* he felt this was the right step for him, open to the possibility that he might be more ambivalent about change than he appeared. But Donal described not only the negative effects he believed his marijuana use was having—increasing forgetfulness, irritability when he couldn't be high— but also a fierce desire to rid himself of what he now viewed as a remnant of a youth that he was determined to leave behind.

So you might imagine Donal's surprise when I told him I didn't want him to try to reduce, much less stop, his marijuana use before we met again. Instead, I asked Donal simply to keep track of *when* he smoked during the coming week and *what was happening*, both around him and inside him, at those times.

In response, Donal revealed that he'd expected to be told that he must immediately commit to complete abstinence, and because he shared the goal of quitting he'd known that he would feel obligated to agree, even though he didn't think such a drastic change was possible. He told me he felt relieved to receive such a different message. At the same time, he believed there was little to learn about his marijuana use, which was just a matter of smoking whenever he had the opportunity, so he was doubtful that the kind of self-observation I was proposing would reveal anything useful. Nonetheless, he was willing to try it.

When he returned the following week, Donal was eager to report what he had discovered: there were, indeed, patterns to when he got high and when his desire to smoke was the strongest. They were connected to his daily schedule. When he first arrived home from work (where he did not get high) the urge was at its most intense, as he felt as though he needed to put down a burden he'd been carrying all day long. The same was true for when he woke up on the weekends—he realized that the prospect of facing a long day alone, without anything external to distract him, filled him with dread, and smoking marijuana was the only way he knew to alleviate that feeling. On the other hand, there were times (in the middle of the evening on workdays, after lunch on weekends) when he found that he was smoking more out of habit, and perhaps boredom, than because he "needed" it.

Thinking about these details and others of his week of self-observation, Donal asked me what to do next. When I wondered whether he could think of a single small step that he felt confident he could take successfully, Donal immediately said he thought he might be able to give up his mid-evening bowl on weeknights. Once again, my response surprised him: I asked Donal to pick a single day during the coming week to skip that mid-evening bowl, paying close attention to what it was like for him to do so, and otherwise to go on smoking as he'd been doing. Although he felt he might be capable of more, once again he agreed.

At our third visit Donal made a tongue-in-cheek "confession": after successfully skipping his mid-evening bowl early in the week, he'd gone ahead and done it again a couple of days later. He'd noticed that on the first evening he'd forgone getting high between arriving at home and getting ready for sleep he'd initially felt bored, but soon found an activity to immerse himself in and didn't think much about getting high until later that night. Having enjoyed his evening, he wanted to see if he could do it again, and he'd had a similar experience the second time around.

Asked how he felt about his week and what he'd learned since starting with me, Donal was very clear: the time he'd taken to observe how his marijuana use fit into his life without trying to change it, and the understanding he had gained, had altered his outlook. He knew that it would remain a challenging process and that he had many more small steps to figure out before he'd get where he wanted to go, but he now believed it was a matter of when, rather than if, he would quit getting high.

A Week of Self-Observation

Although it can feel like "doing nothing," compared with active efforts to change, self-observation has a number of positive effects. As Donal's experience illustrated, self-observation can help reduce the pressure you might be feeling to make progress, which can trigger the old negative cycle of anxiety, avoidance, and self-blame. By giving you a little bit of distance, it can help you see what you are struggling with more objectively or from new angles and become aware of things that are so familiar you hardly notice them anymore. This awareness, in turn, can suggest new ideas and in particular can help you identify "entry points" into change—small, manageable steps that begin to move you in the direction you want to be going and help you build momentum for larger steps down the road.

So I invite you now to embark on a week of self-observation. Like Donal, I'd like you to pay attention to, and keep track of, *when* you engage in the behavior (or are in the situation) you'd like to change and *what is happening* around you and inside you at those times. Importantly, I don't want you to try to change anything this week; just act as you normally would and notice as much as you can: the circumstances you are in, what you are doing, what others are doing, how you are feeling, what you are thinking. At the end of each day, write down what you noticed. Then answer these questions:

- "When did I engage in the behavior (or find myself in the situation) I want to change? What were the circumstances? What was I doing?"
- "How was I feeling at those times? What was I thinking at those times?"

To get a sense of the kinds of things you might discover, look at what Ellie wrote about her week of self-observation before recording your own week in your journal or in the form at *www.guilford.com/zuckoff-forms*.

. . . .

My Week of Self-Observation

Ellie

What were the circumstances? What was I doing?	How was I feeling at those times? What was I thinking at those times?
I started my work days by making sure everyone had their lunches and something for breakfast. I inevitably grabbed a muffin or doughnut to go with my coffee while I did that.	I figured I could have just one thing for myself and I'd make up for the calories by eating light at lunch or dinner. As soon as I bit the muffin, I felt a sense of relaxation.

Twice this week someone brought bagels or pastries for a midmorning snack for the staff. Both times I went and had something.

When I knew there were pastries in the lounge, I told myself that after I finished my first group's notes I would treat myself as a reward. I looked forward to it through the group session, especially because I felt stressed by how much I still had to do.

I keep a bowl of wrapped caramels or chocolates in my office to offer to clients or staff. On stressful days I ate a half dozen or a dozen of those myself.

Sometimes just eating one of my candies helped to calm me and kept me focused on meeting deadlines.

I took a bag lunch to work every day. I usually pack a good lunch, with healthier food, in part because I eat with coworkers. But I also pack chips. This week we had two interns visiting, and I only ate the sandwich during lunch and the rest later at my desk.

I always think my coworkers notice what I'm eating and are thinking critical things about me. If there are women there I don't feel as comfortable with, I save the unhealthy foods until later. I felt self-conscious because of the interns.

One day, I visited the snack machines and bought some cookies and snuck them back to my office in my purse.

I always feel a little ashamed when I do that, but not once I get in my office. Then I just enjoy the cookies! They really help me get through monotonous paperwork.

Several people routinely walk the stairs for exercise, instead of taking the elevator. The same women also go for walks sometimes during lunch and then eat at their desks.

I have a quiet struggle inside every day with the idea that I should walk stairs during lunch or even when I get home. I tell myself that I should, but then I feel uncomfortable when I think of joining the other women and I don't do it. When I get home, I tell myself that I might do it later but that I need to rest and then get to the kitchen to start dinner.

When I got home, after I rested for about 15 minutes, I spent the next

I was feeling tired and hungry but focused on what everybody wanted.

few hours each night in the kitchen preparing supper and cleaning up. Gil and the kids all wanted different things, as always. I grazed on whatever I was fixing. I never sat down to a full meal—I ate standing. Once all the meals were prepared and everyone was eating, I would clean up and then get to work on packing lunches. Afterward, I was tired from being on my feet for hours, so I lay on the couch.

I didn't pay much attention to what I was eating as I was eating it. I just nibbled whatever I could because I was hungry. I do enjoy grazing because it tells me how far I've gotten in cooking everything. By the time I'm packing lunches for the next day I'm really looking forward to getting out of the kitchen. A few times I thought I should exercise, but I told myself maybe tomorrow.

At the end of the night I sat down, watched television, and had different favorite bedtime snacks: cereal, buttered toast, guacamole and chips, ice cream, pudding, a piece of pie or cake or whatever was left over from dessert.

I would feel bad and tell myself I shouldn't be eating like this at this time of night, but then I'd think I'll start tomorrow, or else that trying to lose weight is useless anyway, so why not just enjoy it after working so hard?

On the weekend I shopped for the week and was at home preparing meals and snacks and cooking some meals I could freeze.

I get hungry just looking at all of the food when I'm shopping, so as usual I bought something to eat in the car on the way home.

On Sunday I had coffee and doughnuts at church before the main service; then our family went out for brunch with my in-laws and their families. As usual we all made multiple trips to the buffet and chatted and laughed most of the time we were there.

Sunday brunch is a real highlight for me. It was so nice to spend those hours visiting, relaxing, and eating. I don't feel self-conscious there because several of my sisters-in-law struggle with their weight, too. I feel normal and think to myself, This is all that really matters in life—being with family.

We had a lighter dinner on Sunday. I didn't have to spend much time in the kitchen except to pack lunches and to cook and freeze a stew for later in the week.

By Sunday dinner I'm usually more relaxed because there isn't so much to prepare. I also ate light because as usual I felt bloated from brunch. I told myself that I wouldn't eat so much at next brunch, but I knew I didn't mean it.

REVISITING YOUR PLAN

It's likely that your experience of working toward change has already gotten you thinking about tweaking, adjusting, or adding to your original plan. If you completed the week of self-observation, you might be thinking about more dramatic revisions.

In the sections that follow, I ask you to consider each of the five components of your change plan and decide whether to leave it as is or revise it. Record any revisions in your journal, in the change plan form you completed at *www.guilford.com/zuckoff-forms* or (if you prefer to keep a record of your plan in its original form) in the "Personal Change Plan Revised" form at *www.guilford.com/zuckoff-forms*. As before, give yourself the time to think creatively and be sure that what's in the plan feels right to you.

Also consider, if you haven't already, whether there's information you need to revise your plan for the better or feel more confident. If so, figuring out where to get that information, then thinking about what it means and whether it adds anything valuable to what you already knew, can also be a useful way of strengthening the plan you've developed.

Your Goals for Change Revisited

Please read out loud the changes you wanted to make and ask yourself: "Have my goals changed? Would I answer the question 'What changes do I want to make?' any differently now?" If your answer is yes, then consider the responses of your companions who rewrote or added to their goals in the Personal Change Plan, which appear below, and then revise your own in your change plan record in your journal or the change plan form at *www.guilford.com/zuckoff-forms*.

. . . .

What Changes Do I Want to Make?

Colin

> I not only want to get better at expressing what upsets me to Paul; I want to share myself more openly with him in all ways. I hope that would help him to trust me more fully, too.

Ellie

> The biggest thing the last week taught me was that my weight goal was way too ambitious and I overwhelmed myself. I still want to get back to my prepregnancy weight someday, but I need to start by just trying to change some of my eating patterns because right now losing that much weight sounds about as realistic as a trip to the moon. And the only way I'm going to be able to do anything different is by letting people who love me help me when I need it.

Your Reasons for Change Revisited

Please read out loud your reasons for change and ask yourself: "Have my reasons for working toward change changed? Would I answer the question 'Why do I want to make these changes?' any differently now?" If your answer is yes, then consider the responses of your companions who rewrote or added to their reasons in the Personal Change Plan, which appear below, and then revise your own in your change plan record in your journal or the change plan form at *www.guilford.com/zuckoff-forms*.

Why Do I Want to Make These Changes?

Alec

> I noticed that a main reason was that I felt like I wasn't getting the enjoyment out of life that I could. That is really important to me, and I lost sight of it for a bit. I want to be more than I am, for my family as well as for myself, and I want to have more fun in the process.

Colin

> I want to do this to protect and nurture what I have with Paul but also because I want to learn more about myself and grow as a person. Maybe I thought it was selfish to feel this way, but I don't feel that way now. It would be good for both of us.

Ellie

> I think the way I described my reasons made me feel a little pressured. The truth is, I don't have to do this—life will go on if I don't, Gil will still love me if I don't, and so will God. So I don't have to do this for any of those reasons, but I want to, if that makes sense.

Your Steps Toward Change Revisited

Now that you've had the chance to put the steps you planned to take into action you are in a position to consider whether any of them were unhelpful, and thus can safely be discarded, or less helpful than you'd expected, and thus call for some tweaking. You might also have some new ideas about steps that might work or already have added something to your repertoire of change strategies.

Before you decide about revisions to your steps, consider your companions' revised steps, shown below. Then read your original steps and keep, change, or erase each of them in your change plan record in your journal or in the form at *www.guilford.com/zuckoff-forms.*

. . . .

What Steps Will I Take to Make These Changes?

Alec

Next with Wendy is asking her about a weekly date night. I'll start with just telling her I'd like us to go out and then talk to her about making it a regular thing. I want to start going to the new gym, but I need to figure out how to build it into my daily routine. Jen wants to go in the evening, but that won't work for me. I can get started this weekend and think about when will work during the week. Jim is on this new health track for himself—maybe he'd be up for going to work out together. I'll talk to him about that this week. As for enjoying my life more, we need to make some plans with friends on the weekends, too.

Barbara

It was easier than I'd expected to talk to Steve about doing something together and a little more stressful to talk with him about my feelings. I think once I start opening up that way I'm going to feel a strong pull to have the big conversation, and I want to make sure the timing is right. I feel more ready to do that. But I also need to talk to him about going back to law school, and that's a different conversation. Now I'm thinking I should approach him with this as a possible problem that I want his input on, rather than something I want to do because I am restless and unfulfilled. It's closer to the truth to keep that separate from how I've been feeling in our marriage. So yes, I am going to talk with him about the law school challenge and keep doing the other things I planned to be able to make that happen.

Colin

I will add more focus on self-exploration. I haven't done anything to find a therapist yet, and that needs to be the next thing I put effort into. Maybe

> a therapist would recommend couple counseling, too, and that might move things along further with Paul trusting me. I'm also going to keep looking for a meditation class that fits my schedule.

Dana

> I want to add a step that involves looking around for places where I might live, depending on what school I get into (there's confidence!). And talk to my boss about a part-time option if I stay here in the city. But first, make that call to my parents.

Ellie

> #1 and #4 on my plan need to be greatly expanded. The other steps are good, I think, but I am not really ready for them yet, except for praying for guidance.
>
> 1. The first thing I have to do is talk with Gil and then the whole family about how important it is for me to lose weight and how impossible it will be with our current lifestyle. It's going to be very hard for me to do, because taking care of them means so much to me. But if I continue to spend this much time in the kitchen, I know I will never succeed.
> 2. Then I'm going to ask Gil if he will take over the grocery shopping and see if he will agree to keeping sweets out of the house and shifting over to fruits. Maybe he can take the kids out for ice cream and give me an evening to myself each week.
> 3. I'm going to ask my kids if they want to learn to cook, and I am going to help them to learn how to make healthier meals—this way, I am still helping them, but they will also be helping me. I really like this idea.
> 4. I am also going to have the kids take more responsibility for themselves in the mornings, for breakfast, and for preparing their own lunches. I'll try to do this in a fun way for them, but also let them know that they will be helping me reach a goal. Maybe I'll even give them each a way to cheer me on and figure out rewards for me as I progress. I think I can get them involved in a way that doesn't feel like I'm burdening them. That's important.
> 5. I am going to get a secret support person at work to confide in, and I am going to get rid of my office candy! I'll offer mints instead, or get one of those coffee/tea makers and share that with others. That could be a treat for me, too.
> 6. I'm not going to give up Sunday brunch. But I can give up the third trip to the buffet and make what I take on the second trip last. It's a start.

Your Supports for Change Revisited

Please review the support people you identified and how you hoped they could support you in your efforts at change. Now that you've begun to take action, please ask yourself: "Are there other ways that any of them could help? Are there other people who might also be willing and able to help? If so, who are they, and what could they offer? Anyone I thought might be a positive support but now realize isn't a good fit for that role?"

If your answer is yes, then consider the responses of your companions who rewrote or added to their Supports in the Personal Change Plan, which appear below, and then revise your own in your change plan record in your journal or the change plan form at *www.guilford.com/zuckoff-forms*.

. . . .

Supports for Change

Alec

Whom can I call on for support?	How can they support me?
Jim	If Jim wants to work out together, it would probably help me get into a good routine.

Barbara

Whom can I call on for support?	How can they support me?
My sister	She can tell that something is changing with me, but I haven't gotten into the details with her. I guess I've held back because I don't want her to be too optimistic about things working out perfectly for Steve and me. But even though she'll be happier than is warranted, I still think talking with her could help a lot, so I ought to let her in on what I'm thinking.

Colin

Whom can I call on for support?	How can they support me?
Paul	Ironically, this has felt sort of isolating, because normally he would have been my main support, but now he can't be.

Judy	I've been thinking about asking her to have dinner some night, just to have someone else who cares about both of us to bounce some of this off of.

Dana

Whom can I call on for support?	How can they support me?
A new spiritual community	I want to find a spiritual community wherever I end up going to school. That will be an important support for me when I'm starting over in a new place.

Ellie

Whom can I call on for support?	How can they support me?
Gil	I know Gil would help me in so many more ways if I let him. Not just with practical things, but emotionally. I was thinking I might ask him to join me for my doctor's visit—I'm sure he'd be surprised and happy to do it.
My kids	My kids won't get the emotional importance. But I do think they would enjoy cheering me on and thinking up ways to help, like making up charts or coming up with new activities. I like the idea of involving them, not so much for the actual help, but to give me another focus that feels sort of creative and fun. It will help me to keep things a little "lighter"!
Nancy	My friend Nancy at work is really so sweet and understanding; she's not one to gossip and will always lend a helpful ear to anyone. I'm thinking about confiding in her just so I have a place of respite during my workday—even just to share a cup of tea and a few laughs if I need it. I don't let myself have that out of self-consciousness, and my stress relievers or breaks are too often just sweets!

Your Hurdles and How You'll Get Past Them Revisited

By now you may already have encountered some of the hurdles you antici-pated. If you have, the question to ask yourself is "How well did my planned solutions work?" If you managed those challenges well, it's fine to stay with the solutions you've identified; if not, this is your chance to come up with some alternatives.

Of course, you might also have run into some hurdles that caught you by surprise. Again, ask yourself: "How well did I manage them? What are the alternatives for dealing with any hurdles that knocked me off my stride?"

Consider the responses of your companions who rewrote, added to, or erased hurdles and solutions in their Personal Change Plan, which appear below, and then revise your own in your change plan record in your journal or the change plan form at *www.guilford.com/zuckoff-forms*.

. . . .

Hurdles and Solutions

Alec

What hurdles could arise?	What will I do to overcome them?
Scheduling workout time.	I should be fine going to the gym in the morning if Jim can't join me. I'll start out with a couple of days a week to gradually establish a new routine. And if I have a busy week, I'll just take a run at home.

Barbara

What hurdles could arise?	What will I do to overcome them?
If Steve doesn't support me going back to law school?	This would be a big hurdle. I guess I would need to listen to his concerns, consider them, and see if we could work something out together. It is so interesting that just as I write this, I realize that working this out together is not how I have approached this so far, but I have this feeling of hope that we probably could if we tried.

Colin

What hurdles could arise?	What will I do to overcome them?
Can't find a good therapist.	I do worry about this, because I am picky and do not want to talk with someone who is going to start to blame me. I think I'd sense that pretty quickly. I would keep looking until I found a good match.

Ellie

What hurdles could arise?	What will I do to overcome them?
1. My biggest hurdle is that so many of the foods I love and turn to for stress relief and pleasure are high-calorie, high-fat, high-bad-for-you. I look forward to them all through the day but especially at the end of the day.	1. This will probably be my hardest challenge. I can keep the candies out of my office and probably even resist the snack machine at work. And spending less time in the kitchen will help, too. But what will I do when I crave something tasty? Fruit will do as a substitute sometimes. Maybe I can find some lo-cal ice cream treats and things like that. But I need to think harder about things I can do to de-stress.
2. My other hurdle is getting over my reluctance to ask for help. I could get mad at myself if I cheat or frustrated if I don't see progress and then send the message that it's no longer such a big deal for me.	2. Maybe connecting in little ways at work could help with this. Like texting or one of those cell phone games you can play with someone else might keep me from feeling too isolated. It might help with stress at work, too! I will tell Gil about this and maybe my sister.

- -

Signs of Success

A final step, as you prepare to put your revised plan into action, is to iden-tify signs that will tell you your plan is working. Although some goals can be reached quickly, the changes you're working toward may be more com-plex and it may take some time to get where you're going. When working toward more distant goals it's important to be able to recognize markers along the way that will confirm you're on the right track. This will not only guide your decisions about sticking with your plan or revising it further—it will also help you sustain your motivation to keep working at change over the long term.

So please ask yourself this question: "How will I know that my change plan is working?" Consider your companions' responses, shown below, and then record your answers in your journal or in the form at *www.guilford. com/zuckoff-forms*.

How Will I Know That My Plan Is Working?

Alec

If things keep getting better with Wendy. We start being able to enjoy ourselves again, laughing and joking around, without a feeling of tension between us. Feeling more like we're on the same side. When I don't have to think about skipping that last drink or making them last. Having that old energy in the morning like I used to have. Looking forward to coming home at the end of the day. My spare tire starts to shrink. Feeling like I'm getting what I want out of life and like I'm putting my best effort into it.

Barbara

I'll know my plan for changing my relationship with Steve is working when we are talking about real things and not just making conversation. When I look at him and feel desire. When I see him looking at me with desire. When he says something that surprises me and I laugh spontaneously. I'll know my plan to restart my career is working when I have a timeline for when I'm going to start school—once that's in place I know it will take on a life of its own.

Colin

The biggest sign will be that I don't have to work so hard to control my anger—I won't get angry as often, and when I do, I'll be able to contain it, and if I need to express it to Paul I'll be able to do it in a way that doesn't scare or hurt him. I'll start to see Paul look at me the way he used to, or take my hand, or rub my back spontaneously. Or he'll initiate spending time together doing something new. I'll feel less on eggshells around him. I'll be able to relax enough to show mild irritation without worrying that he's going to get upset. We'll be able to have some fun again. We can invite friends over again for dinner parties. We can make love. We can plan for our future together. And I'll be able to continue my own personal exploration without feeling like something else is at stake while I'm doing it.

Dana

> I already know it's working. All I have to do is keep going.

Ellie

> Dropping a few pounds will be a good sign. But I've done that before. What will really show me that it's working is if I'm going about it in a different way. When I talk with my secret work support person, when there is no more candy in my office for weeks, when I find things that I genuinely look forward to other than food, when I take some creative steps with my kids, and most important, when I talk with Gil about what I feel I need.

THE WAY FORWARD

The way forward from here will look a lot like the way you've come so far. From this point on, your process of change will involve continuing to act on your current plan and revisiting it regularly to decide whether and in what ways it needs to be revised again. The absence of the signs you've just identified will alert you to the need to plot a different course—perhaps by making minor adjustments or perhaps through more substantial changes.

At the same time, it's also valuable to keep one eye on the further horizon. By this I mean not just achieving your change goals—ending the habit you want to eliminate or establishing the one you want to cultivate; removing yourself from the situation you want to get out of or ensconcing yourself in one you wanted to get into; changing the pattern that interfered with your relationships or with getting what you want out of life—but sustaining the changes that you've made and continuing to move toward the life goals that matter most to you. In the final chapter I offer guidance on increasing your likelihood of success in both of these pursuits.

• • • • 9 • • • •

The Far Side of Change

Change involves entering the unfamiliar and having it become familiar. The process by which this happens is often gradual, although sometimes it's punctuated by sudden shifts that only in retrospect appear to have been inevitable.

When I was in college, I decided to take voice lessons. I'd always enjoyed singing, but I knew my vocal limitations meant that my enjoyment was not always shared as enthusiastically as I would have liked by those who were listening to me.

I did the exercises my teacher assigned and worked hard to incorporate the techniques I was learning. I changed the way I breathed and how I formed sounds with my mouth; I relaxed my tongue and firmed up my diaphragm. And as the weeks and then months passed, I noticed a change: I now sounded worse than I had before I started and felt awkward and self-conscious instead of confident and natural.

Worried that I had gone from an adequate singer to one who nobody could possibly tolerate, I spoke with my teacher and wondered whether I wouldn't be better off going back to my previous mediocrity. When he assured me I was on the right track, I agreed to stick with it a little bit longer despite my misgivings.

And then, about 6 months into my voice lessons, something magical happened. When I opened my mouth to sing, a sound came out that I had never heard before: rich and vibrant. Excited, I told my voice teacher what had happened at our next lesson. Of course, he said—your body has been learning a new way of producing sound; it just needed some time for the muscles to develop and to be able to do what your brain told it to do.

When you start to act in a way that's different from the way you've always acted or you enter a new situation (or leave one that you know well), it's almost inevitable that it will feel strange or awkward—"not you." As you give up the security of who you were while not yet having become who you're going to be, the temptation may be strong to seek out the solid ground of the familiar. Sometimes you make the adjustment little by little; sometimes an extended period of feeling as though you're spinning your wheels is followed by a surprising moment of gaining traction. But as every person who's learned to ride a bike or drive a car (or sing with good technique), or who's moved to a new town or begun a new relationship, knows, making it to the far side of change brings rewards that can't be gained any other way.

PATHWAYS TO CHANGE

Although everyone who makes a change has the experience of entering the unfamiliar, in other respects peoples' pathways through change can vary based on the kind of change they're making as well as its difficulty and complexity. Following are four pathways you might find yourself on as you work to implement your plan, with some guidance on how to maximize your chances of carrying your change process through to successful completion.

The Decision Is the Change

For some kinds of dilemmas, the most difficult part is making the decision between competing options; once that decision has been made, the way ahead and the steps to be taken are clear. A person who decides, for example, to donate an organ to a loved one who needs it to survive will have to go through many procedures before the donation surgery takes place; yet the path ahead is clearly laid out for him, and reaching his goal requires only that he follow that path to its end. Similarly, a person who decides to accept a job offer does not need to make an elaborate plan for carrying out her decision; once the acceptance has been conveyed there will be steps to take (informing her current employer, saying good-bye to coworkers, going through the human resources process at her new place of work), but all of them are likely to follow relatively routinely.

If, like Dana, this describes the pathway you are on, then you need little more guidance from me. I describe Dana's pathway through change to illustrate what being on this pathway is like and perhaps to highlight some ways in which she was able to ensure a successful outcome by following her heart, trusting her own judgment, and dealing with the practical issues in front of her.

Dana's Pathway: "I Can Hardly Believe How Far I've Come"

More, even, than all the practical steps she took to embark on her career as a teacher, the key moment in Dana's process of change was the phone call she made to her parents, asking them to dinner so she could tell them about her plans for the future. Before she could finish her sentence, her mother knew what she was going to say; rather than having to persuade them that she was making a responsible choice, the dinner turned into a planning session for how everyone would manage the changes her new direction would bring about, and finally a celebration of her joy in her new future. Serious and reserved at the start, her father wanted to be sure that she had thought her decision through, and he raised a number of concerns that Dana viewed as legitimate. But as he heard how thoroughly she had done her research and how much she already knew about the financial aspects of the decision, she could see his growing respect and then feel his pride in the daughter he had raised. In Dana's words:

> "It makes me chuckle now to think about how nervous I was to talk with my parents about my decision to apply to grad school. I'll never forget that night, though, because it was so satisfying to talk through everything as three adults. And the best part was that they respected my desire to do something meaningful, and I could tell them that I was only trying to be the person they raised me to be."

The actual process of becoming a graduate student brought some challenges. After she aced the GRE, Dana's top choice accepted her but offered no financial assistance, whereas her second choice offered an assistantship that would allow her to forgo working outside of school. Efforts at negotiation were followed by several frazzled nights of wrestling with the options, until she realized that her second choice was now her first and she accepted their offer—a decision she would not regret. When she gave her notice, her employer surprised her with a going-away party, which allowed her to leave with a feeling of good will and closure. Her friends, as expected, were nothing but excited for her, and they made sure she had a chance to celebrate before starting her new life as a graduate student.

From there it was a whirlwind of finding a place to live, starting classes, and getting reacclimated to being a student and living "a little bit poor again" so as to leave her savings untouched. And, in some ways most important to her, she joined a church where she felt accepted and at home from the moment she got there. As Dana contemplates her progress in her process of change:

> "I'm so excited for this year and next year and each year after that! I feel like my old self again . . . no, actually, I feel more like myself than I ever have. When I look back on this past year, I can hardly believe how far I've come."

Riding the Momentum

At first, the decision that Barbara believed herself to be leaning toward but unable to accept—to leave her husband—would have appeared to lead her into a pathway of the sort that Dana was on. If she decided to leave, she would certainly have faced further decisions and challenges—where to live and how to support herself financially being the most obvious— but it's unlikely that any of them would have been a source of significant ambivalence or that she would have found herself struggling to maintain her commitment to carrying them through. She might well have needed to find sources of both practical and emotional support, but not to develop a detailed plan for how carry out her decision.

However, once Barbara realized that she did not want to leave Steve, but that she wanted to rebuild her life with him (as well as an independent career), the uncertainties she faced—in how to approach Steve and how to determine her best and most viable career options—put her on a different path. In that situation she did need to develop a step-by-step plan that she could follow for each of her goals and revisit and revise that plan as new aspects of her situation emerged. The choice she made required her to change long-standing behaviors—talking more openly and honestly with Steve about her real feelings and wishes, for example—that would be challenging for her at first and that she would have to become gradually more comfortable with.

Similarly, the intertwined goals that emerged from Alec's resolution of his ambivalence—to cut back on his drinking, reestablish a close and mutually respectful relationship with his wife, and start paying more attention to his own well-being, all in the service of restoring balance and enjoying his life more—required not just an initial plan but a process of revisiting, revising, and recommitting himself to carrying his plans forward over time. Like Barbara, Alec faced a situation in which some important influences on his ability to achieve his goals—for example, how Wendy would respond to the change in the timing of his return home on weeknights, as well as the condition he came home in—were outside his control. And also like Barbara, some of the behaviors he'd have to engage in—choosing to drink less and communicating differently with Wendy around areas of disagreement between them—would take some time before they became "second nature" and he could confidently assume that his actions would match his intentions.

At the same time, Alec and Barbara found themselves carried forward on their change pathways by the success they experienced as they began to implement their plans. Although they had to make adjustments along the way, both found that their initial plan put them on track for success and that the key to sustaining change was to keep their reasons for pursuing their goals foremost in their minds while enjoying the fruits of their labors. If this also describes the path you are on, you may find it helpful to follow the progress made by Alec and Barbara and to implement some of the strategies they used to ensure your own success.

Alec's Pathway: "I Don't Even Feel Like Hanging Out at the Bar Anymore"

As Alec kept coming home from work sober and early most nights, the tension between Wendy and him continued to diminish, and this, in turn, motivated him to keep to his plan. He could see that Wendy was pleasantly surprised when he suggested they have an evening out together on an upcoming weekend when Jen would be at a slumber party, and even more so when he told her that he thought it would be good for them to do this sort of thing regularly. It was she who then suggested they turn some of these dates into nights out with friends, and his enthusiastic agreement was met with a bigger smile from her than he'd seen in some time.

Going to the gym was iffy at first. He went regularly for a few weeks, then got busy at work and slowly tapered off. He asked Jim about joining him, but their schedules conflicted, although later they would occasionally go for a run together. Soon he noticed that he wasn't feeling quite as energetic as he had been, and he started to act more irritable with Wendy, even though he hadn't returned to late nights out.

When Alec and Wendy started to bicker again, and one night he came home later than usual to find her with tears in her eyes, Alec was tempted to revert to old habits. But this time he did something different:

> "When she told me I was late and smelled like alcohol, I wanted to defend myself, remind her of how many times I'd come home early, tell her she's never satisfied. But when I looked at her, I saw she wasn't really angry or disrespecting me—she was scared. And then I didn't

feel like arguing. I just wanted to let her know that she didn't need to worry and that I wasn't about to throw away our progress."

So the next day Alec spoke with his senior account manager about the challenges he was facing balancing home and work. His manager replied that he'd had a similar problem in the past and worked it out by shifting his hours. As Alec had also begun negotiations for the promotion he'd hesitated about, he added that he was reluctant to increase his travel time and be away from his family more. It turned out that his bosses recognized how strong an employee Alec was, and they modified his position into one focused on training and supervising newer sales reps. Once he made the transition, Alec was able to arrange his schedule to work out in the mornings and had fewer evenings out entertaining clients, reducing his stress and making Wendy very happy in the process.

When Alec and Wendy went out for their anniversary some months later, he was struck by the difference from their last anniversary dinner. He surprised her with a new necklace—the kind of gift he'd have given her earlier in their marriage but not in recent years. He recalled the distance between them a year earlier and knew that their easy intimacy that night had a lot to do with their having resumed their long-dormant sex life not long before. That had only happened once Alec realized that the resentment Wendy had built up during the years he came home late and drank too much wasn't going to dissipate just from his changing his behavior; he'd needed to show her he understood how much he'd hurt her and recognize that she'd been questioning the viability of their marriage as a result.

As Alec reflects back on the changes of the prior year he feels optimistic:

> "The kicker to all this is that I don't even feel like hanging out at the bar anymore. I'm just fine having one drink on most nights. It doesn't faze me, and if anything work is going better than it was. My last doctor's visit was a lot more pleasant, too. I've lost some weight, and he didn't mention alcohol. And my blood pressure is better. If I can finally get myself out to the garage to start working on the Camaro, I think I'll be all set."

Barbara's Pathway: "I Could Never Have Anticipated Where This Path Would Lead"

When Barbara finally began to talk with Steve about her career aspirations, she did not get the response she expected. That he was completely supportive did not surprise her. But when he admitted one evening that he'd been worried that he was losing his desire for her because he could only see her as the mother of their children, she was taken aback. He went on to confess that he was "out of the habit" of looking at her sexually and had been for some time. So, when Barbara had shared her ambitions with him, he suddenly started seeing her in a different light—as he had when they were first dating and she was full of energy and enthusiasm for the career she intended to have. He was, he said, "excited by [her] excitement."

Barbara never told Steve that she had initially worried that their marriage was all but over, and as far as she knew Steve never had those thoughts himself. But she did let him know that she had felt similarly to the way he described. After that, they were able to talk much more easily, and Barbara could feel that he wanted them to get to know each other again, in a new way, just as she did. As their conversations deepened and she felt her marriage beginning to be restored, she reflected on what had helped her negotiate some treacherous waters:

> "I feel so grateful to my sister, especially, and my friends for helping me get through this. When I finally told them what I'd been thinking they slowed me down and let me bounce things off them before I tried to talk it through with Steve. I could have made a mess of it if I had just dumped all this on him without taking the time I needed to sort out my feelings."

After doing some more research, Barbara decided to obtain a master of public health degree instead of returning to law school. This both seemed to her a more manageable course of action and better suited to the possible career directions she realized she wanted to pursue. Accepted into a program near her home, she attended an orientation where she found a blend of traditional and nontraditional students like her and began to think about how she could best put her talents and energy to good use.

> "This feels like a whole new life for me. Steve and I feel much closer to each other now. I would not say that we are burning with passion, but that doesn't matter much to me anymore, at least the way it did before. It feels like I think a couple should feel after so many years of marriage: deeper and more personal. I respect him more than I did even when I married him, and I think the feeling is mutual. We are fortunate to have each other. And when I look back at how I started this whole process, I realize that I could never have anticipated where this path would lead."

The Need to Persevere

For people whose change goals—such as losing significant amounts of weight, quitting smoking, or overcoming dependence on alcohol or drugs—require not just a change in particular behaviors, but broader changes in lifestyle and patterns of interaction with others, sustaining change and continuing on track toward their goals often requires more than the willingness to stay focused on change and ride the momentum of their initial efforts. The needs to reconsider goals to make them more achievable, actively persist in making concrete changes, cope with unexpected hurdles, and regularly call on sources of support place more demands on those who are on this path and make success appear much less certain than it can appear in the pathways I've previously described. Nonetheless, for those who are willing and able not only to persevere but to remain open to revisiting and revising their change plans and finding ways to be kind to themselves as they do so, this pathway can also end in successful change.

If this is the path you find yourself on, you may find useful guidance in a description of how Ellie sustained her motivation and commitment and went a long way toward achieving her change goals.

Ellie's Pathway: "Sometimes I Look Forward to Time with Friends Even More than Dessert!"

Even after she revised her original weight loss goal and her steps toward change following her week of self-observation, reducing the pressure she'd inadvertently put on herself and making her change process seem more manageable, Ellie continued to feel shaky about her prospects. Talking with Gil about how the family's patterns would have to change to give her any chance of success was a big step that paid off handsomely—not only was Gil right alongside her, ready to help (as deep down she knew he would be), but he offered to be the one to talk to the kids as well, which she knew he could do more easily and (she had to admit) effectively than she could. The kids rose to the occasion; with a little grumbling from the 9-year-old (who was going to miss his cookies) but huzzahs from her health-conscious vegetarian 15-year-old, all were willing to clear out the junk food and make way for fruits and rice cakes. The change made it easier for Ellie to go into the kitchen, although she still found herself spending more time there than she thought was good for her. Her friend Nancy was similarly enthusiastic about helping her at work: she made it her job to anticipate situations that could be challenging, like the day everyone took the agency's receptionist to lunch for Secretary's Day and she was able to influence the group to go to a restaurant with healthy options.

Ellie began by weighing herself weekly, and when she'd lost 3 pounds after the first week and another 2 after the second she was very encouraged. But when she got on the scale the following week and saw it tick upward she felt all her motivation draining away. Although she told herself that she had to be patient, and that she'd done really well by making those initial changes, she didn't tell anyone what she saw on the scale that morning. Soon, despite the pep talks she gave herself, she found herself avoiding Nancy at work and even snuck down to the snack machines a couple of times. Ellie describes what it was like:

> "I felt so terrible inside, it's hard to put it into words. I bought a candy bar and ate it in the ladies' room, in a stall. I could feel my mind racing, and it was almost like an argument with myself: 'You're a failure; no matter what you do, you're never going to lose this weight,' versus 'Hang in there, the scale is not a measure of your worth or even your progress.'"

When Ellie got home that day, she went straight to the bedroom; Gil, knowing something was not right, followed. Although she tried to hide how she was feeling as she'd always done, this time she started to cry as she told him, "It's no use, I'll always be fat." Gil held her while she cried and went on to tell him about the scale and the candy bars. He told her to rest for a while, and that he loved her, and went downstairs.

After falling asleep for a while—a luxury she never allowed herself in the evening, when there was a family to be fed—Ellie went downstairs to find dinner on the table. In tears again, though this time happy ones, she sat as the kids told her how they'd helped their father prepare it, and her 15-year-old jumped up to bring her the special healthy plate they'd made for her.

Later, Gil asked Ellie what they could do to give her more support and help her keep the inevitable bumps from turning into crises. Thinking together, they agreed that staying off the scale would be a good idea, and Ellie stuck to this decision thereafter, weighing herself monthly instead. When she told him how great it felt not to have to make dinner that night, Gil agreed to work with the kids to keep Ellie out of the kitchen at least a couple of nights a week. He also asked if she wanted to join a bowling league with him or take a ballroom dancing class, which she had wanted him to do years ago. Knowing how he really felt about dancing, she gratefully took him up on the bowling idea, which not only got her moving a bit but brought a new group of friends.

Ellie also took up a suggestion from her oldest; instead of waiting for weight milestones to buy herself new clothes, she started getting her hair or nails done regularly and shopping for one new item—clothing, handbag, even socks—no matter what she thought was happening with her weight. Ellie found that doing these things kept her on track without being caught up in the numbers on the scale and helped to take the month-to-month variations in how much weight she lost in stride. She even allowed herself to get a massage for the first time.

She also continued to allow herself some comfort foods, just not as often and not as much. At work, she and Nancy began taking their afternoon break together, sometimes going for a walk or just having tea. She also took up crocheting again, which prompted several women at work to ask her to teach them how to do it, too. Once a week, Ellie and her "apprentices" now crochet on their break, and Ellie finds herself doing it whenever she needs something to do with her hands, especially when she feels nervous or stressed. Her projects included a sweater for her daughter and a scarf for Nancy, to show appreciation for all her help.

Ellie feels more at peace with herself, while still aware of the work yet to be done:

> "So far, I have lost 17 pounds. That's enough for me to feel differently about myself, even though I still have a long way to go. But that's not the only thing making me feel better about me. I feel closer to God, more like I am bringing out my best self. I'm doing things that are a little uncomfortable for me but help me in the long run. I've started to believe that a little bit of success is not the same as failure. I'm realizing that letting people in my life help me makes them feel as good as helping them makes me feel. And sometimes I look forward to time with friends even more than dessert!"

Temporary Setbacks

This is the most precarious pathway for people who embark on change. For those who begin to make progress toward their goals, and then experience one or more setbacks, some feelings of frustration and even discouragement are inevitable. Yet these feelings need not result in hopelessness or abandonment of the change process. If setbacks are understood for what they are—temporary (and completely normal) reversions to behavior that is highly familiar and thus readily available, most often in times of stress or (paradoxically, it might seem) relaxation (when one has let down one's guard and allowed oneself to respond "instinctively")—then the path to change is easily recognizable and not very difficult to resume.

The precariousness of this pathway, ironically, is caused not by the setback itself, but by a particular way of interpreting it. When a person who has achieved abstinence from alcohol or drugs briefly returns to drinking or using, or a former smoker gives in to the urge for a cigarette, or a person who has stopped screaming, threatening, or hitting others lashes out in a moment of violent anger, the feeling of failure—and the belief that he has just proven to himself that he will "always" end up back at square one, or that she has demonstrated to significant others that she can never really be trusted—can set in motion an especially powerful version of the "terrible triad" of anxiety, avoidance, and self-blame (with its toxic cousin, debilitating shame). The results are highly predictable—the urge to relieve the anxiety by any means available, including the very behavior (smoking, drinking, drug use, raging) that the person was trying to change; the defensive impulse to minimize the need for change and rationalize accepting defeat; and the continuing justification for self-punishment (name-calling, self-humiliation, depriving oneself of the chance of achieving the goals that matter most) that the return to the old, familiar behavior provides.

If you have landed on the setback pathway, I hope you'll read Colin's story and find within it the help you need to head off the terrible triad. As you'll see, after his initial progress Colin found himself faced with a setback that tempted him to give up on himself and the goals that meant so much to him. The ways in which he managed to resist that temptation, learn from his setback instead of letting it hurt him, and recommit to his process of change may provide you with useful guidance in meeting the challenge you find yourself facing.

Colin's Pathway: "I Have to Take Better Care of My Own Feelings"

During the first few months Colin continued to feel as though things were progressing with Paul and with gaining control over his anger. Continuing the steps he'd already begun to take, he also started a meditation class and found that it was helpful not only for managing his emotions but also for getting more in touch with what was going on inside him. He began to make plans for his new studio and took more time to work on his art at home. He also tried to focus on Paul in a different way, working to understand his feelings and know him more deeply. He managed not to be reactive, taking a break or a walk when he felt tension rising or noticed he was sounding irritable or frustrated.

At the same time, Colin found himself wondering how long it would be before he felt the old feelings of closeness with Paul or when their time together would start to feel more comfortable and spontaneous. Moments when it seemed as though this was beginning were quickly followed by a feeling of distance between them, a sense that Paul was keeping him intentionally at arm's length.

One night, after dinner together, Colin felt that familiar longing and decided the time was right to take a chance. So he sat next to Paul on the sofa and started to pull him closer. Here is how Colin describes what happened next:

> "He smiled at me and nicely took my hand off him and said that it was not a good time. My disappointment must have shown on my face, because he said, gently, that after all we've been through together he didn't want to mess things up by going too quickly. Without thinking, I said that 'too quickly' for him felt like an eternity for me. Well, that was evidently not the right thing to say, because he turned cold and curt and said that if I wasn't satisfied, then maybe this wasn't going to work out. Part of me knew that he was feeling hurt and defensive, but my mind started to race, and before I could think about deep breaths or walking away or anything else I blew up. I shouted that this was the sort of passive–aggressive crap that had started all of this and blamed him for being impossible to get close to. In a rage, I yelled who knows how many more hurtful things, and he yelled back, too. Then I stormed out."

Colin stayed at a hotel that night. He returned the next day, but it seemed to him that things with Paul had gone all the way back to square one or even worse. They avoided each other coming and going, and Colin spent the next week trying to figure out how to end the relationship once and for all. He felt horrible about everything—himself, Paul, all of the effort they'd put in. He told himself that it was pointless and they were just mismatched. He veered between thoughts that Paul was too fragile and unwilling to look at his own part in their problems and, most of the time, thinking of himself as hopeless and berating himself for being so stupid as to mess up the best thing he'd ever had. He waited, miserably, for Paul to tell him that he was done.

Finally, when he couldn't stand it anymore, Colin went over to Judy's house. At first he acted as though he was doing fine, even after she told him that she knew what had happened. But after dinner he told her that he didn't know which way to turn, that he was feeling terrible about himself and dreading word from Paul that he was going to leave. He told her that he had finally blown up one too many times and that he couldn't blame Paul for having had it.

Colin could see a look of seriousness and confusion on Judy's face. She said that Paul did not want to leave and that he loved Colin deeply. She said that, while he was upset by this most recent outburst, he did not feel as hurt as he had in the past because he had been keeping a safe distance emotionally. She said that he had expected this to happen eventually and that while his distance was necessary for his own protection, he knew it was hard for Colin.

After his long conversation with Judy the situation began to become clearer for Colin. He understood that Paul's distance was a way of preserving the relationship while gradually building trust. Still, he knew that he would need more help to tolerate the pace of rebuilding that Paul needed to maintain, so he made the inquiries to find a therapist he'd been putting off. He kept in mind something Judy had said: that if he kept his focus on himself, and did not look to Paul too anxiously for signs of progress, he might find those signs to be more forthcoming.

When Colin had his first session with his new therapist, whom he felt comfortable with immediately, he told Paul, emphasizing that he intended to keep working on himself. Paul's response, that he was working on things, too, gave Colin the first feeling of hope he'd had since before the setback (as his therapist referred to it). Paul also told him that he did not think they had gone all the way back to square one and that he could feel the difference that Colin's efforts were making. Bloodied but unbowed, Colin's thoughts realistically reflected both the challenges and the possibilities ahead:

> "I don't know that I believed all of what Paul said, but it felt good to hear it, and to talk with him calmly yet with real feeling. Letting him hear me, without shouting at him—I haven't been very good at that, and I need to get better. I was right when I realized that I need to pay more attention to myself, but in the sense that I have to take better care of my own feelings instead of expecting Paul to do it for me. It sounds strange, but it feels like I have to let go of Paul a little for us to become closer in a new way."

SELF-REWARDS AS SELF-CARE

Whichever path your change process is following, a key to sustaining change is to make sure your efforts to improve your life are not all work and no play. As we've seen, sometimes the changes we make bring their own inherent rewards. But especially when the pathway you are on includes gradual change that requires maximal effort, or setbacks that you must face and overcome, building in opportunities to feel good and to affirm yourself for the hard work you are doing constitutes effective self-care and can help you maintain the motivation required to see your efforts through to the end.

Sometimes, when change is a struggle, people can begin to question whether they actually deserve to feel good or reward themselves. So before I ask you to think about the kind of rewards you'd most welcome, I'd like to help you remember why you're worthy of them.

Please think about the best compliment you ever received and ask yourself these questions:

- "Who gave it to me?"
- "What made it so memorable and so valuable to me?"
- "What did it tell me about myself that I didn't know or perhaps didn't appreciate as much until someone recognized it?"

At different times, Colin and Ellie—both engaged in change processes that require persistence and resilience in the face of setbacks; one feeling down on himself, the other temperamentally reluctant to think about nice things she could do for herself—found the prospect of self-rewards difficult to contemplate. You can see their responses to these questions below before writing your own in your journal or in the form at *www.guilford.com/zuckoff-forms*.

. . . .

The Best Compliment I Ever Received

Colin

Compliments on my art are nice, but they don't usually stick with me because I'm always focused on the next piece. But there is one compliment that meant a lot to me. This little girl who lived in our apartment building used to come over to watch me paint. I liked her because she was kind of quirky for a 7-year-old. I would talk with her while I worked, about all sorts of stuff, or I just listened to her stories. One day I ran into her mother, and she told me they were moving and she wanted to thank me for spending time with Lori. She'd told her parents that I helped her deal with the kids at school and with anticipating her move. She said I'd given Lori self-confidence by letting her know she was unique and special in how she thought about the world. I always remember that moment, how it made me feel special that I could give her that, just by being myself with her.

Ellie

I have always had a hard time taking compliments directly. When my bowling average started to go up, I got so many compliments from others in our league. The attention was hard to take! And then the women I taught to crochet told me what a great teacher I am and how my pieces are so lovely, too. I had several people ask me if they could commission me for presents. I wanted to tell them it was nothing, but I admit it did feel good. But the best compliment ever? It has to be the one I got from my youngest last week, when she told me that she wants to be just like me when she grows up—"You can do anything, Mommy, and my friends tell me that I have the nicest and most fun mom, and you're so beautiful, too!" She is my greatest fan.

- -

I hope that you are now ready to consider rewarding yourself and think about how you might want to do so. As with the other components of your change plan, rewards are not "one size fits all"; what's rewarding for one person might not feel especially rewarding for another. At the same time, there are some useful guidelines you can follow.

A large body of research by psychologist Edward L. Deci and colleagues[1] shows that the effects of rewards vary based on whether the person receiving the reward feels *controlled* by it. When we do something for its own sake, because of the pleasure or satisfaction we get from doing it—whether playing a game, pursuing a hobby, doing something nice for someone we love, or anything else—we don't need or expect to receive a reward for it. In fact, being offered a reward can even make us like doing whatever we were doing *less* than before. Imagine how you might feel if, in response to surprising your friend with a gift, your friend offered you money as a reward for your thoughtfulness. You would probably protest: "I didn't bring you this gift because I wanted a reward! I brought it to you because I wanted to do something nice for you!" And the pleasure you felt at your gesture would likely be greatly diminished, as your sense of yourself as acting generously of your own free will gets tainted by the implication that your action was motivated by the desire to get something back.

On the other hand, rewards that give us *feedback* on our performance—that tell us how well we are doing when we're working to accomplish something—are usually not experienced as controlling; instead, they're usually experienced as giving us useful information for gauging our progress at something we are internally motivated to do. That's why students, under the right circumstances—when they are interested in the subject they're studying and feel challenged by their assignments—can feel even more

---

[1]Deci, E. L., with Flaste, R. (1996). *Why we do what we do: Understanding self-motivation.* New York: Penguin Books.

motivated to learn when they receive a grade that affirms their hard work and tells them they have mastered the material.

So the key to effective self-reward is not only to find something to give yourself that feels genuinely rewarding. It's also to avoid trying to control yourself with the promise of an external reward ("You have to work for one more hour before you have a treat"), running the risk of triggering *reactance* at your effort to control your own behavior ("I can have a treat right now if I want!")—but instead to find nice things to do for yourself that aren't contingent on completing any particular action but that affirm your continuing efforts at change and appreciatively acknowledge that what you are doing requires courage and fortitude.

With these guidelines in mind, please ask yourself: "How can I reward myself for my continuing efforts at change?"

Colin and Ellie both ultimately found building in self-rewards a valuable addition to their change plans. Here's what they came up with, to consider before you record your own in your journal or in the form at *www.guilford.com/zuckoff-forms*.

- -

How Can I Reward Myself for My Continuing Efforts at Change?

Colin

I've been going out more with the other artists at the gallery where I started to show my work. I also decided to take classes in areas that I have wanted to develop in myself—starting with an advanced French class to reestablish my fluency. But I also learned from my therapist that I need to <u>add</u> helpful behaviors rather than just trying to stop the problem behavior. So Paul and I have started a new ritual of surprising each other every other week. Sometimes it's taking the other one somewhere new; sometimes it's a story from our past we haven't told each other, or a new book, or whatever. We always present it in an envelope, with a card that explains why we chose it. (This was my creative version of my therapist's suggestion that we go on a date each week—boring!) I like knowing that he's thinking about us, and it helps to have this to look forward to. And there's no pressure on pleasing the other person, because the focus is on what we want to share from and for ourselves.

Ellie

The rewards I've been getting from reaching out to others have been very fulfilling. I've started to look forward to treating myself to a new outfit when

> there's an event to go to. I've also been noticing the good feeling I get when I realize I can move my body more easily, and it has me thinking about fun things I can do in the future, like bicycling, swimming, or maybe even dancing. Thinking like that gives me a good feeling inside.

THE WAY FORWARD: REFLECTING ON YOUR EXPERIENCE OF CHANGE

As this book comes to a close, I hope you have found within it the means not only to resolve the ambivalence you were struggling with when you first read the line "Something in your life has become an issue for you" but also to see, hear, and accept yourself in a different way and to feel capable of making the changes you want to make when you're ready to make them. Ideally, your experience of working through this book could serve as a template for how you might take on future dilemmas—because the one thing I'm certain of is that you, like every other person, will face your share of them in the course of your life.

So I'd like to ask you to reflect on your experience one last time. Looking back to the beginning, and thinking about all you've read, written, and thought about since, please ask yourself: "What do I know now that I didn't know before? What have I learned that I'd like to take with me?" Use your journal or the form at *www.guilford.com/zuckoff-forms* to record your thoughts.

We end with your companions' answers to these final questions.

What Have I Learned from My Process of Change?

Alec

> One thing I learned is that it doesn't have to be "me versus you" when there's conflict in a marriage. We got stuck in a tug of war when we really wanted the same things. It took time for me to see that Wendy was not against me when she was upset about my drinking; she just cared about me and missed us having good times together and wanted to be treated with respect, just like I did. The other thing is that things get better when I'm taking care of myself. It's easy to get caught up in work and stress when it's all you're focusing on. I was forgetting to make time to live my life and keep some balance.

Barbara

I learned at the very beginning that it's important to accept what you feel to find out what it means and where the feelings may take you. I was so afraid of my feelings, I tried to stifle them or impulsively do something to get rid of them. This helped me slow down and not expect to know the right answer for everything right away. I also learned that other people are not just one thing, but if you see them that way that's all they'll be with you. I only saw Steve as static and unexciting because I stopped paying attention! I always knew how to set a goal and work to achieve it, but I didn't really know how to give myself or other people the space to change from the inside. That's a valuable lesson and one I plan to hold on to.

Colin

I'm definitely still learning. I know now that I can accept that I've hurt someone and need to change without it meaning that I'm "wrong" and he's "right." That just because something doesn't seem harmful to me it doesn't mean that it can't hurt someone else. That I don't have to turn the person I love into the enemy because he's telling me he doesn't like what I'm doing. But I've also realized I can express myself in ways other than through my art and people will listen—at least people who care about me. This sounds ridiculous now, but I thought I was done growing as a person before this all started, like I was who I was and that was the end of the story. Now I know that change is hard, but it's possible.

Dana

I don't think I learned so much as I remembered things I already knew deep inside but lost track of for a time. When something really matters to me, and it's where I feel I'm being guided spiritually, nothing is really going to stand in my way. I was trying to fight my true calling for a long time, but it wasn't working and never really could. And once I realized what needed to be done, all I had to do was trust in my own good judgment and sense of responsibility to carry me through. It's easy to lose your way, I think, when life demands start to take over, but I am so glad that I found my path again, and I know it is the right one for me.

Ellie

More than anything, I learned that I cannot keep telling myself that even though I "know" I should be willing to let the people in my life help me, I just don't feel right doing it. I am not some special case who is supposed to give to others and not cherish herself. I have needs and desires just like everyone else. It's still hard for me to accept this fully, but I'm getting there.

The History and Science of Motivational Interviewing

Motivational interviewing (MI) was the brainchild of William R. Miller, PhD, currently Emeritus Distinguished Professor of Psychology and Psychiatry at the University of New Mexico. (Well known for his modesty and lack of pretension, when I congratulated him on being awarded emeritus status upon his retirement, Bill—as everyone calls him—dryly replied that the literal meaning of the term is "of former merit.")

As a graduate student in psychology in the 1970s, when psychology departments in the United States commonly maintained rigid and even hostile boundaries between competing theories and orientations, Bill had the good fortune to be exposed at the University of Oregon to both the "client-centered" (later, "person-centered") counseling approach developed by leading humanistic psychologist Carl Rogers (*On Becoming a Person, A Way of Being*) and extended by his student Thomas Gordon (*Parent Effectiveness Training*), on the one hand, and the "cognitive-behavioral" therapy approach founded on the conditioning theories of B. F. Skinner (*Science and Human Behavior, About Behaviorism*) and social learning theory, in the form of Gerald R. Patterson's behavioral family therapy (*Families: Applications of Social Learning to Family Life*), on the other. (One of Bill's teachers, Hal Arkowitz, PhD, went on to become a central figure in the "psychotherapy integration" movement that has tried to break down those barriers and bring together the best of all available approaches; in a neat reversal, Hal later became trained in MI and has made important contributions to the literature on MI as an author and editor.)

It's no exaggeration to say that MI represents an integration of two seemingly irreconcilable counseling approaches. Bill's ability to pull together aspects of these and other social psychological theories derived from his fundamentally pragmatic way of thinking: his interest was not in whether the theories were compatible (which, arguably, they're not), but whether each approach had something valuable to offer to counselors and other clinicians in their day-to-day efforts to help their clients.

It was during a clinical placement at a Veterans Administration (VA) alcohol rehabilitation center that Bill's first inklings of what would become MI arose. At that time, the dominant approach to counseling people with alcohol problems was the "confrontation of denial" model. Similar to what you might have seen on the TV show *Intervention* or countless other popular portrayals, "alcoholics" were believed to suffer from the symptom of denial, which purportedly made it impossible for them to recognize the damage that their drinking was doing; the only way to help them, it was believed, was to "break through" that denial by any means necessary and force them to see the truth of their behavior. For Bill, though (as for many of us who later came to MI through our work with people with substance use disorders), treating anyone this way—"alcoholic" or not—ran counter to all that he had learned about helping relationships, not to mention his personal values of compassion and respect for others. So Bill began talking to his clients at the VA the same way he'd talked to the clients he'd worked with before—trying to understand their way of seeing themselves and the world and, on the basis of that understanding, to help them identify behaviors they were willing to work toward changing and then to help them make those changes.

It was not, however, until a serendipitous sabbatical in Bergen, Norway, and a clinical practicum he led with a group of young Norwegian psychologists, that the method of MI was formulated. As Bill has recounted many times, these bright young clinicians peppered him with questions about why he took this or that approach with a client he was talking to or why he recommended a particular intervention to his supervisees. Forced for the first time to put his underlying assumptions and the implicit rules that had been guiding his practice into words, Bill was inspired to draft an article that was published in shortened form in 1983 under the title "Motivational Interviewing with Problem Drinkers." (In 2008, in celebration of the 25th anniversary of the founding of MI, I had the privilege, as editor of the newsletter of the Motivational Interviewing Network of Trainers [MINT], *MINT Bulletin*, to publish the original uncut manuscript of that paper in facsimile form; you can find it, free of charge, at *www.motivationalinterviewing.org/sites/default/files/MINTBulletin14.2.1.pdf*).

Looking back at that article more than 30 years later, it's remarkable to see how much of our current understanding of MI could already be found in its first presentation. Also present was what I think of as Bill's "magpie" tendency to pick and choose the best bits of other approaches to establish and shape his own creation—prominently, the theory of cognitive dissonance. ("Cognitive dissonance" as an explanation for why helping people focus on the gap between their behavior and their attitudes could motivate them to change behavior later gave way to the language of "discrepancy" between where the person was and where he wanted to be, or who the person was and who she wanted to be, and theories of self-regulation and goal attainment.)

Bill's original article was little noticed in the United States in the years following its publication, but that was not the case in the United Kingdom. (The journal that published the article was based in Britain.) There, and elsewhere in Europe, psychologists began to explore the use of MI principles in work with people with alcohol and drug use disorders, as well as with people with eating disorders, which in many ways resemble addictive behaviors. When he learned about the spread of MI into clinical practice, Bill felt a bit embarrassed; he was a researcher, and here he had promulgated a counseling approach for which he had no research evidence, only his own clinical experience. So he set out to correct this omission, embarking on a series of studies that would establish the beginnings of MI's status as an evidence-based intervention.

But before I discuss these studies, I need to tell you about the second founding moment of what we now know as MI. In 1989, while visiting Australia, Bill met a British (by way of South Africa) psychologist named Stephen Rollnick, PhD, who told Bill that he had come across the original article on MI, begun practicing the method it described, and then started training others in the approach as well. Recognizing a kindred spirit, Bill invited Steve (as he is universally known) to coauthor a book in which they would present an expanded and updated version of MI. The publication of *Motivational Interviewing: Preparing People to Change Addictive Behavior* by The Guilford Press in 1991 brought MI to a much wider audience, especially in the United States, than it had reached previously. It also introduced a broader variety of theoretical sources and clinical practices into MI, from Sharon and Jack Brehm's theory of reactance (discussed in Chapter 2), to the decision counseling of Irving Janis, to Albert Bandura's research on self-efficacy (discussed in Chapter 5), to Daryl Bem's self-perception theory (discussed in the First Interlude), and more. And, crucially, it placed *ambivalence* at the center of the context in which MI could be most helpful and even transformative for people struggling with change.

From this point forward, Bill and Steve collaborated in developing the theory and practice of MI, through two more editions of their basic MI text from The Guilford Press: *Motivational Interviewing: Preparing People for Change* (2002), which recognized and furthered the expansion of MI's reach beyond addiction problems; and *Motivational Interviewing: Helping People Change* (2013), which acknowledged that MI had applications beyond "behavior change" to other kinds of changes that people might struggle with. In these books and numerous articles published in the interim, Bill and Steve developed and refined their understanding of the "spirit" of MI (introduced in the Prelude), the conceptual structure through which it operates (originally five, and then four, "principles," now "four processes" of Engaging, Focusing, Evoking, and Planning—as well as key constructs including importance, confidence, and commitment), and the counseling strategies and techniques that MI practitioners could use to help people resolve ambivalence. Having found a professional home in a medical school, Steve—now Honorary Distinguished Professor in the Cochrane School of Primary Care and Public Health, School of Medicine, Cardiff University, Wales—also led the expansion of MI into healthcare settings with several books[1] and studies of MI provided in those settings by nurses and others not trained as professional counselors.

In the late 1980s Bill conducted the first study of MI by testing whether a brief intervention, consisting of a thorough assessment followed by a single 60- to 90-minute MI counseling session incorporating personalized feedback of the assessment results, could reduce drinking problems in problem drinkers who were not interested in formal treatment.[2] This initial study was followed by several that tested MI's usefulness as a prelude to formal treatment, for adults entering an outpatient alcohol treatment program,[3] for adolescents entering an outpatient addiction treatment program,[4] and for adults entering inpatient alcohol rehabilitation.[5] When each of these studies demonstrated positive effects for MI, other researchers began to show interest—most prominently, the developers of what would end up as the largest psychotherapy study ever done, which compared several approaches to counseling people with alcohol dependence as outpatients or following inpatient detoxification: The National Institute of Alcohol Abuse and Alcoholism (NIAAA) multisite study known as Project MATCH.

The goal of Project MATCH was, as the name implied, to discover whether different counseling approaches were better "matches" for different kinds of people with alcohol problems. As it turned out, despite enormous

---

[1]Rollnick, S., Mason, P. G., & Butler, C. C. (1999). *Health behavior change: A guide for practitioners.* London: Churchill Livingstone; Rollnick, S., Miller, W. R., & Butler, C. C. (2008). *Motivational interviewing in health care: Helping patients change behavior.* New York: Guilford Press.

[2]Miller, W. R., Sovereign, R. G., & Krege, B. (1988). Motivational interviewing with problem drinkers: II. The drinker's check-up as a preventive intervention. *Behavioural Psychotherapy, 16,* 251–268.

[3]Bien, T. H., Miller, W. R., & Boroughs, J. M. (1993). Motivational interviewing with alcohol outpatients. *Behavioural and Cognitive Psychotherapy, 21,* 347–356.

[4]Aubrey, L. L. (1998). *Motivational interviewing with adolescents presenting for outpatient substance abuse treatment.* Unpublished doctoral dissertation, University of New Mexico.

[5]Brown, J. M., & Miller, W. R. (1993). Impact of motivational interviewing on participation and outcome in residential alcoholism treatment. *Psychology of Addictive Behaviors, 7,* 211–218.

efforts to specify and measure a large number of potential matching variables, little was learned in that regard. (People who were angrier benefitted more from MI than from the other approaches; people whose social networks were heavily alcohol-focused did better with a 12-step, AA-based counseling model.) However, what seemed remarkable to many was that MI, in the form of a four-session intervention labeled Motivational Enhancement Therapy (MET),[6] was as effective overall as 12 sessions of cognitive-behavioral therapy or 12-step facilitation in helping clients change their use of alcohol.

The success of MET in Project MATCH, combined with the fact that MI could be offered as a brief (one- to four-session) counseling intervention, was the primary source of the explosion of interest in MI among researchers studying how to help people with a wide variety of problems in a wide variety of settings. To date, MI has been tested in more than 250 "randomized controlled trials" (RCTs), the kind of study (considered the "gold standard" in medical research as well as in tests of psychotherapy approaches) that can determine whether a treatment works at all (by comparing it with a "placebo," or a treatment that is not expected to have any effect) or whether it works as well as or better than other bona fide treatments. It has been provided by psychologists, psychiatrists, social workers, counselors, nurses, physicians, dentists, nutritionists, criminal justice professionals, and others and shown positive effects in contexts as varied as anxiety disorders, asthma, brain injury, cardiovascular health, dentistry, diabetes care, dieting, domestic violence, dual (psychiatric and substance use) disorders, eating disorders, emergency department trauma prevention, exercise, family therapy, gambling, HIV/AIDS, medication adherence, mental health treatment engagement, obesity, pain treatment, probation and parole, sexual risk reduction, and tobacco use. In a series of "meta-analyses," in which researchers combine the results of many studies to assess the overall effectiveness of a treatment approach, MI has consistently been shown to be an effective brief intervention—although, like all treatment interventions, not always effective in every setting, and with variable effects.

The question of whether MI "works," then, is generally accepted as settled: It does. But RCTs cannot answer another, equally important question: *Why* and *how* does MI work? (And what's the difference between the times MI works and the times when it doesn't?) Although the theory of MI provided a plausible explanation for its effectiveness, research was needed to open the "black box" called MI and look inside it to determine its effective ingredients or "mechanisms of action"—that is, the specific *causes* of MI's effects.

One way to do this is to compare two slightly different versions of MI and see whether one version works better than another—which would mean

---

[6] Miller, W. R., Zweben, A., DiClemente, C. C., & Rychtarik, R. G. (1992). *Motivational enhancement therapy manual* (Project MATCH Monograph Series, Vol. 2). Washington, DC: National Institute on Alcohol Abuse and Alcoholism.

that the strategies or techniques used in the superior version were at least part of the source of MI's impact. Bill conducted the first study of this type,[7] comparing two assessment-and-feedback interventions: one in which the feedback was given in the style of MI (empathic, nonconfrontational) and the other in which the same feedback was given in a more confrontational style. As predicted, those who received the empathic, nonconfrontational feedback showed much better reductions in their alcohol use—and the amount of confrontation in any counseling session was a good predictor of *more* drinking by the client a full year later. Similarly, a comparison of traditional client-centered counseling with MI showed that its effectiveness was a product of more than just its client-centered components.[8]

Later, a more detailed and revelatory approach to understanding what is happening during MI sessions—involving "coding" or labeling what clients and/or counselors say during MI sessions and looking for the effects of these speech acts on what clients do after the counseling is finished—produced a landmark study that inaugurated the important category of MI *quantitative process research* studies. In a collaboration with psycholinguist Paul Amrhein, PhD, Bill and colleagues coded clients' "change talk" (discussed in the First Interlude) in MI sessions and showed that clients who expressed more commitment were more likely to change their use of drugs following counseling.[9] In the years that followed, MI researcher (and practitioner) Theresa Moyers, PhD, developed methods for coding not only client speech but also counselor speech, demonstrating in a series of important studies[10] that MI practitioners' *interpersonal skillfulness* (i.e., empathy, collaboration, and support for clients' autonomy) and *technical skillfulness* (i.e., use of MI-consistent techniques) both made it more likely that clients would engage in change talk during MI

---

[7]Miller, W. R., Benefield, R. G., & Tonigan, J. S. (1993). Enhancing motivation for change in problem drinking: A controlled comparison of two therapist styles. *Journal of Consulting and Clinical Psychology, 61,* 455–461.

[8]Sellman, J. D., MacEwan, I. K., Deering, D. D., & Adamson, S. J. (2007). A comparison of motivational interviewing with non-directive counselling. In G. Tober & D. Raistrick (Eds.), *Motivational dialogue: Preparing addiction professionals for motivational interviewing practice* (pp. 137–150). New York: Routledge.

[9]Amrhein, P. C., Miller, W. R., Yahne, C. E., Palmer, M., & Fulcher, L. (2003). Client commitment language during motivational interviewing predicts drug use outcomes. *Journal of Consulting and Clinical Psychology, 71,* 862–878.

[10]Moyers, T. B., & Martin, T. (2006). Therapist influence on client language during motivational interviewing sessions. *Journal of Substance Abuse Treatment, 30,* 245–251; Moyers, T. B., Martin, T., Houck, J. M., Christopher, P. J., & Tonigan, J. S. (2009). From in-session behaviors to drinking outcomes: A causal chain for motivational interviewing. *Journal of Consulting and Clinical Psychology, 77,* 1113–1124; Moyers, T. B., Miller, W. R., & Hendrickson, S. M. (2005). How does motivational interviewing work? Therapist interpersonal skill predicts client involvement within motivational interviewing sessions. *Journal of Consulting and Clinical Psychology, 73,* 590–598.

sessions,[11] and that clients who engaged in more change talk in general (not only commitment talk) were more likely to make changes after the counseling was finished. Other researchers have also investigated various components of MI practice, looking to elucidate which of those components are necessary for effective MI practice and which are not; affirmation, in particular, appears to play an especially potent role.[12]

Despite the remarkably large volume of research studies that have been published on MI, in many respects we are still only scratching the surface in understanding what makes MI the effective counseling approach that it is, and ultimately how to do MI better for the sake of people who are stuck in ambivalence and looking for help in resolving it. Over the next decade or more, we expect to learn not only from the kinds of studies I've described here but also from new methods, including neuroimaging techniques that have already begun to hint at the brain activity of someone who is participating in a motivational interview, and thus about MI's effects at the neurological level.[13] New applications of MI—for such purposes as helping prospective living organ donors to resolve residual ambivalence about donation, which has been shown to result in poorer postsurgical outcomes in the altruistic people who give the gift of life to another who needs it[14]—have begun to emerge and show promise. Members of the MI community—centered on MINT, an international

---

[11]See also: Borsari, B., Apodaca, T. R., Jackson, K. M., Mastroleo, N. R., Magill, M., Barnett, N. P., et al. (2014, August 11). In-session processes of brief motivational interventions in two trials with mandated college students. *Journal of Consulting and Clinical Psychology*. Advance online publication. *http://dx.doi.org/10.1037/a0037635*; Magill, M., Gaume, J., Apodaca, T. R., Walthers, J., Mastroleo, N. R., Borsari, B., et al. (2014). The technical hypothesis of motivational interviewing: A meta-analysis of MI's key causal model. *Journal of Consulting and Clinical Psychology, 82*, 973–983.

[12]Apodaca, T. R., Borsari, B., & Magill, M. (2014, June). Which individual clinician behaviors elicit or suppress client change talk and sustain talk? Paper presented in plenary session at the 4th International Conference on Motivational Interviewing, Amsterdam, Netherlands.

[13]Feldstein Ewing, S. W., Filbey, F. M., Hendershot, C., McEachern, A., & Hutchison, K. E. (2011). A proposed model of the neurobiological mechanisms underlying psychosocial alcohol interventions: The example of motivational interviewing. *Journal of Studies on Alcohol and Drugs, 72*, 903–916; Feldstein Ewing, S. W., Filbey, F. M., Sabbineni, A., Chandler, L. D., & Hutchison, K. E. (2011). How psychosocial alcohol interventions work: A preliminary look at what fMRI can tell us. *Alcoholism: Clinical and Experimental Research, 35*(4), 643–651; Feldstein Ewing, S. W., McEachern, A. D., Yezhuvath, U., Bryan, A. D., Hutchison, K. E., & Filbey, F. M. (2013). Integrating brain and behavior: Evaluating adolescents' response to a cannabis intervention. *Psychology of Addictive Behaviors, 27*, 510–525; Feldstein Ewing, S. W., Yezhuvath, U., Houck, J. M., & Filbey, F. M. (2014). Brain-based origins of change language: A beginning. *Addictive Behaviors, 39*, 1904–1910.

[14]Dew, M. A., DiMartini, A. F., DeVito Dabbs, A. J., Zuckoff, A., Tan, H. P., McNulty, M. L., et al. (2013). Preventive intervention for living donor psychosocial outcomes: Feasibility and efficacy in a randomized controlled trial. *American Journal of Transplantation, 13*, 2672–2684.

organization of more than 1,200 MI trainers, practitioners, and researchers in more than 35 countries and 20 different languages, on whose Board of Directors I served from 2008 to 2014 (the last 2 years as chairman)—have been publishing books as part of The Guilford Press series on the use of MI with a variety of populations and problems,[15] as well as with other publishers.[16] There is also a growing body of research on how to help practitioners learn to conduct MI more skillfully and the beginnings of research on how to help organizations adopt MI in order to improve their counseling services.

From the perspective of an MI practitioner, trainer, and researcher, the chance to contribute to the ongoing growth of a relatively young, vibrant, and evolving approach to counseling provides as much professional satisfaction as one could hope for. And from the perspective of the general public, there is every reason to expect that the continuing development in our understanding of how to provide, and teach others to provide, MI will bring increasing benefit to those who feel trapped in dilemmas they cannot resolve.

---

[15]Arkowitz, H., Westra, H. A., Miller, W. R., & Rollnick, S. (2015). *Motivational interviewing in the treatment of psychological problems* (2nd ed.). New York: Guilford Press; Hohman, H. (2013). *Motivational interviewing in social work practice.* New York: Guilford Press; Naar-King, S., & Suarez, M. (2010). *Motivational interviewing with adolescents and young adults.* New York: Guilford Press; Wagner, C. C., & Ingersoll, K. S. (2013). *Motivational interviewing in groups.* New York: Guilford Press; Walters, S. T., & Baer, J. S. (2005). *Talking with college students about alcohol: Motivational strategies for reducing abuse.* New York: Guilford Press; Westra, H. A. (2012). *Motivational interviewing in the treatment of anxiety.* New York: Guilford Press.

[16]Douaihy, A., Kelly, T. M., & Gold, M. A. (2014). *Motivational interviewing: A guide for medical trainees.* New York: Oxford University Press; Schumacher, J. A., & Madson, M. B. (2014). *Fundamentals of motivational interviewing: Tips and strategies addressing common clinical challenges.* New York: Oxford University Press.

Resources

For help with your dilemma from a psychotherapist, there is currently no central place where you can go to find a counselor who provides motivational interviewing specifically.

To find a qualified psychotherapist in your area:

- **United States and Canada:** The American Psychological Association's "Psychologist Locator," at *http://locator.apa.org*, allows you to search by location, gender, ages served, specialization, languages spoken, and other characteristics of a psychologist that might be important to you.

- **United Kingdom:** The British Psychological Society's "Directory of Chartered Psychologists," at *www.bps.org.uk/bpslegacy/dep*, allows you to seach by location, ages served, presenting issue, and languages in addition to English.

- **Ireland:** The Psychological Society of Ireland's "Psychologist Online Register," at *www.psychologicalsociety.ie/find-a-psychologist*, allows you to search by location and discipline.

- **Australia:** The Australian Psychological Society's "Find a Psychologist," at *www.psychology.org.au*, allows you to search by location and the issue you're concerned with.

- **New Zealand:** The New Zealand Psychological Society's "Find a Psychologist," at *www.psychology.org.nz*, allows you to search by location, ages served, and psychology work area.

To learn more about MI, MINT's website, at *www.motivationalinterviewing.org*, provides free information, articles, and other resources on MI and the research that supports it. In addition, MINT's online, open access journal, *Motivational Interviewing: Training, Research, Implementation, Practice* can be found at *www.mitrip. org*. If you're a practitioner, *Motivational Interviewing: Helping People Change* (3rd ed.; New York: Guilford Press, 2013), by William R. Miller and Stephen Rollnick, the founders of MI, is the basic text on the approach. David B. Rosengren's *Building Motivational Interviewing Skills: A Practitioner Workbook* (New York: Guilford Press, 2009) provides practical, step-by-step guidance for learning how to provide MI with clients.

Readings that complement, supplement, or build on the principles and practices described in this book include the following:

• *Changing for Good: A Revolutionary Six-Stage Program for Overcoming Bad Habits and Moving Your Life Positively Forward* (reprint ed.; New York: William Morrow Paperbacks, 2007): James O. Prochaska, John Norcross, and Carlo DiClemente provide guidance on how to become ready for healthy change and take action to achieve it. Their approach, based on their scientifically supported "transtheoretical" model of behavior change, is a cousin to motivational interviewing.

• *Changeology: 5 Steps to Realizing Your Goals and Resolutions* (New York: Simon & Schuster, 2012): John C. Norcross, Kristin Loberg, and Jonathan Norcross present a condensed and simplified program also based on the transtheoretical model. Like *Changing for Good*, it is most helpful for people who know what they want to change but are having difficulty accomplishing it.

• *Self-Compassion: The Proven Power of Being Kind to Yourself* (New York: William Morrow, 2011): Kristin Neff provides a practical approach to reducing self-criticism. In drawing a contrast between self-compassion and self-esteem, she overemphasizes the negative ways that self-esteem can be pursued (through comparing ourselves with others and judging ourselves superior) and neglects the positive ways in which it can be cultivated (through genuine accomplishment and earning the esteem of others we care about). But the exercises in this book can help you increase your self-acceptance and self-care and decrease the effects of the terrible triad of ambivalence. This book is especially suitable for readers with a strong spiritual outlook.

• *Why We Do What We Do: Understanding Self-Motivation* (New York: Penguin Books, 1996): Edward L. Deci (with Richard Flaste) provides an accessible account of his theory of self-determination, explaining how *support for autonomy* can help us pursue courses of action we feel "intrinsically motivated" for and why making such choices makes us more likely to succeed at change.

• *The Lost Art of Listening: How Learning to Listen Can Improve Relationships* (2nd ed.; New York: Guilford Press, 2009): Many of the lessons taught by Michael P. Nichols about listening to others can also be applied to listening to ourselves, a crucial component of the motivational interviewing approach to helping people resolve ambivalence about change.

Index

A Way of Being (Book), 249
Ability talk, 86–87, 126. *See also* Confidence for change
About Behaviorism (book), 249
Acceptance, 9, 61, 62–63, 65, 68, 70, 71, 82. *See also* Self-acceptance
of self, 62, 82
Accurate empathy. See Empathy
Activation talk, 87, 166
Activities
A Difficult Challenge I Overcame (Chapter 5), 131–134
A Look Back (Second Interlude), 162–164
Brainstorming (Chapter 7), 195–198
Committing to Your Plan (Chapter 7), 211
Confidence for Chapter 5, 135–136
How Am I Already Living Out the Values That Matter Most to Me? (Chapter 6), 153–155
How Can I Reward Myself for My Continuing Efforts at Change? (Chapter 9), 246–247
How Can My Successes and Strengths Help Me with the Changes I Want to Make? (Chapter 7), 192–193
How Will I Know That My Plan Is Working? (Chapter 8), 228–230
How Would I Like to Be Living Out My Core Values More Fully? How Is My Current Behavior or Situation Keeping Me from Doing That? (Chapter 6), 156–158
Hurdles and Solutions (Chapter 7), 208–211
Hurdles and Solutions Revisited (Chapter 8), 227–228
Imagining Change (Second Interlude), 168–169

Imagine I Had to Decide Right Now (Chapter 2), 39–40
Importance and Confidence (Chapter 1), 30–33
Importance and Confidence for the First Interlude, 89–92
Importance for Chapter 4, 115–117
Learning from Past Efforts to Make These Changes (Chapter 7), 190–192
Looking Back from an Ideal Future (Chapter 7), 197–198
Marking Change Talk and Sustain Talk (Chapter 4), 95–97
Marking Change Talk and Sustain Talk (Chapter 5), 121–122
More Reasons for Change (Chapter 4), 111–113
More Reasons for Keeping Things the Same (Chapter 4), 101
My Ability to Change (Chapter 5), 126–131
My Ambivalence and Theirs (Chapter 1), 33–34
My Personal Values (Chapter 6), 143–147
My Week of Self-Observation (Chapter 8), 218–220
Positive Qualities You Might Possess (Chapter 3), 72–73
Pressure from Others about My Dilemma (Chapter 2), 43–45
Pressure on Myself about My Dilemma (Chapter 2), 53–56
Pressure on Myself in Other Areas (Chapter 2), 48–52
Readiness to Change (Second Interlude), 165–166
Readiness Redux for the Second Interlude, 172

Activities (cont.)
Reasons for Change (Chapter 4), 103–111
Reasons for Keeping Things the Same (Chapter 4), 99–101
Reflecting on Acceptance and Compassion Received and Given (Chapter 3), 68–70
Reflecting on Choosing My Positive Qualities (Chapter 3), 73–74
Reflecting on Giving Myself Acceptance (Chapter 3), 70–71
Reflecting on My Most Characteristic Positive Qualities (Chapter 3), 80–81
Reflecting on My Values Exploration (Chapter 6), 160
Reflecting on the Impact of Pressure from Others (Chapter 2), 45–46
Reflecting on Pressure I Put on Myself about My Dilemma (Chapter 2), 56–57
Reflecting on Pressure I Put on Myself in Other Areas of My Life (Chapter 2), 52–53
Reflecting on the Importance of Change (Chapter 4), 114–115
Reflecting on the Importance of Keeping Things the Same (Chapter 4), 102–103
Supports for Change (Chapter 7), 205–207
Supports for Change Revisited (Chapter 8), 225–226
The Best Compliment I Ever Received (Chapter 9), 244–245
The Need Being Met by the Status Quo (Second Interlude), 171–172
The Positive Qualities That Are Most Characteristic of Me (Chapter 3), 74–76
The Story of My Ambivalence (Chapter 1), 27–28
The Values That Matter Most to Me (Chapter 6), 148–153
What Changes Do I Want to Make (Chapter 7)?, 183–184
What Changes Do I Want to Make? Revisited (Chapter 8), 221–222
What Changes Would I Have to Make to Live Out My Values More Fully? (Chapter 6), 158–159
What Do I Want My Life to be Like? (Chapter 7), 185–187
What Has Gone Well So Far? (Chapter 7), 213–215
What Have I Already Been Thinking about Doing? (Chapter 7), 189–190
What Have I Learned from My Process of Change?, 247–248
What I'd Most Want to Hear from People Who Have Pressured Me (Chapter 3), 63–65
What I'd Say to Help Someone in My Shoes Feel Accepted and Understood (Chapter 3), 65–68
What Might Change Cost Me? (Second Interlude), 170–171

What Steps Will I Take to Make These Changes? (Chapter 7), 199–203
What Steps Will I Take to Make These Changes? Revisited (Chapter 8), 223–224
What Would I Need to Feel More Confident? (Chapter 5), 137–138
When Two of My Positive Qualities Showed Themselves (Chapter 3), 76–80
Why Did I Choose That Number Rather Than a Lower One (Chapter 4)?, 93–95
Why Did I Choose That Number Rather Than a Lower One (Chapter 5)?, 119–121
Why Do I Want to Make These Changes? (Chapter 7), 187–188
Why Do I Want to Make These Changes? Revisited (Chapter 8), 222
Why Haven't I Given Up? (Chapter 5), 125
Advice, 3–7, 65, 68, 175–178
Affirmation, 9, 89, 244, 246, 255
Alcohol use (drinking), 2, 4, 6, 14–15, 21, 36, 59–60, 87, 124, 179, 184, 185, 204, 234–236, 238, 241, 250, 251, 252–253, 254
Alec (companion), 14–15, 21–22, 31, 43, 46, 49, 52, 53, 56, 63–64, 66, 69, 70, 74, 75, 77, 80–81, 86, 90, 92, 94, 96, 103–105, 112, 114, 116, 120, 121, 126–127, 131–132, 135, 137, 147, 148–149, 153–154, 156, 158, 160, 162, 165, 166, 183, 185–186, 187, 189, 193, 195–196, 197–198, 200, 205, 208, 211, 214, 215, 222, 223, 225, 227, 229, 234–236, 247
Ambivalence about change
anxiety and, 25–27, 40, 46–47, 61, 82, 241
aspects of, 23–27
avoidance of, 25–27, 82, 241
confidence and, 29–30, 33, 89
contradiction and, 27
control and, 37–39
decisional balance and, 101
defined, 7, 13–14
emotions and, 23–24
importance and, 28–29, 30, 33, 89
internal debate and, 24–27, 101
misery of, 42
motivational interviewing and, 251–252, 255, 258
negative judgment and, 37, 39
pathways through, 9
readiness and, 43
resolving, 7, 23–27, 28, 34, 43, 47, 68, 82, 86, 89, 93, 99, 117, 118, 141–142, 161, 167–168, 211, 234, 247, 252, 258
scale analogy, 61
self-blame and, 25–27, 61, 82, 241
shame and, 241
stuck(ness) in, 13, 22–27, 34, 36, 40, 71, 88, 142–143, 156, 255
status quo side of, 98–103
terrible triad of, 25–27, 82, 241, 258
values and, 141–143, 156
varieties of, 13–14, 21–22

Anger, 17–18, 22, 24, 26, 36, 39, 40, 46, 71, 87, 216, 241
Anxiety, 20, 25–27, 40, 46–47, 61, 82, 168, 217, 241
Anxiety disorders, 253
Amrhein, Paul, 254
Arkowitz, Hal, 249
Autonomy
    defined, 9
    motivational interviewing and, 9, 254
    support for, 38, 62, 254, 258
    control and, 37–39, 62

Bandura, Albert, 118, 251
Barbara (companion), 15–17, 21–22, 31–32, 44, 46, 49, 52, 53–54, 57, 64, 66, 69, 70, 74, 75, 77–78, 81, 86, 90, 92, 94, 96, 105–106, 112, 114, 116, 120, 122, 127–128, 132–133, 135, 137, 147, 149–150, 154, 157, 158–159, 160, 163, 165, 166, 183, 186, 187, 189–190, 191, 193, 196, 198, 200–201, 205, 205–206, 209, 211, 214, 215, 223, 225, 227, 229, 234–235, 236–237, 248
Beckett, Samuel, 213
Bem, Daryl J., 85, 251
Bergen, Norway, 250
Bobblehead effect, 5, 41
Brainstorming, 194–199
Brehem, Jack, 251
Brehem, Sharon, 251
Buyer's remorse, 42

Career decision, 2, 5, 13, 16, 18–20, 23, 32, 87, 141, 232–234, 236–237
Changeology: 5 Steps to Realizing Your Goals and Resolutions (book), 258
Changing for Good (book), 258
Change goals, 182–184, 185, 188, 189, 203, 211, 230, 238
Change Plan. *See* Personal Change Plan
Change talk, 121, 122, 126, 254–255
    ability talk in, 86–87, 126
    activation talk in, 87, 166
    ambivalence and, 88
    balance of, 98, 123
    commitment talk in, 87, 166, 254, 255
    confidence and, 121, 135
    defined, 86
    desire talk in, 86, 98
    identifying, 95–98, 102–103, 121–122, 125
    importance and, 103
    in motivational interviewing, 254–255
    mobilizing, 86–88, 166–167
    need talk in, 87
    preparatory, 86–88, 166
    reasons talk in, 87, 111
    taking steps talk in, 166
Client-centered counseling, 249, 254
Cognitive dissonance, 251
Cognitive-behavioral therapy, 249, 253

Colin (companion), 17–18, 22, 32, 44, 46, 50, 52, 54–55, 57, 64, 67, 69, 70, 74, 75–76, 78–79, 81, 86, 90–91, 92, 94–95, 96–97, 99–103, 106–108, 113, 114–115, 116, 120, 122, 128–129, 133, 136, 137–138, 147, 150–151, 154, 157, 159, 160, 163, 165, 166, 183, 186, 187, 190, 192, 193, 196–197, 198, 201–202, 206, 209–210, 211, 214–215, 221, 222, 223–224, 225–226, 228, 229, 241–243, 244, 246, 248
Collaboration, 254. *See also* Partnership
Commitment (to change), 30, 39, 87, 166, 167, 180, 211, 215, 234, 238, 252
Commitment talk, 87, 166, 254, 255
Compassion, 62–63, 65, 68, 70–71, 82, 250. *See also* Self-compassion
    in MI spirit, 9
Confidence for change, 8, 22, 28–30, 34, 117, 118–138, 161, 166
    as a dimension of motivation for change, 30, 34, 89
    exploring, 126–131
    importance of the status quo and, 98–99
    importance of change and, 123–124
    in motivational interviewing, 252
    past success and, 131–134
    rating, 30–33, 89–92, 124, 135–136
    self-efficacy and, 118–119
    strengths and, 131–134
Confrontation of denial, 250
Control, 37, 39, 47,48, 57, 62, 88, 143, 246
Core values, 141–143, 148, 156, 185. *See also* Values

Dana (companion), 18–20, 22, 32, 44–45, 46, 50–51, 52, 55, 57, 64, 67, 69, 70, 74, 76, 79–80, 81, 86, 91, 92, 95, 97, 108–109, 113, 115, 116, 120, 122, 129–130, 133–134, 136, 138, 147, 151–152, 155, 157, 159, 160, 163, 165, 166, 183, 186, 188, 190, 202, 206, 210, 211, 215, 224, 226, 230, 232–234, 248
Deci, Edward L., 245, 258
Decisional balance, 101
Defensiveness, 42
Denial, 30, 36, 250
Desire talk, 86, 92, 98, 102
Di Clemente, Carlo C., 258
Discrepancy, 251
Donal (case example), 124–125, 216–218

EARS (acronym), 86, 89, 115, 135
    defined, 89
Ellie (companion), 20–21, 22, 32–33, 45, 46, 51–52, 55–56, 57, 65, 67–68, 69, 70–71, 74, 76, 80, 81, 86, 91, 92, 95, 97, 109–111, 113, 115, 116–117, 121, 122, 123, 125, 130–131, 134, 136, 138, 147, 152–153, 155, 158, 159, 160, 164, 165–166, 168–172, 184, 186–187, 188, 190, 193, 197, 198, 202–203, 207, 210–211, 215, 218–220, 222, 224, 226, 228, 230, 238–240, 245, 246–247, 248

Empathy, 254
Envisioning change, 166, 170
Exercise, 2, 20, 86, 253
　　case example, 199

Failure
　　effect on confidence, 30, 118, 188, 204
　　learning from, 191–192
　　terrible triad of ambivalence and, 241
*Families: Applications of Social Learning to Family
　　Life* (book), 249
Finding your way to change, how to use, 9
Feedback, rewards and, 245
Flaste, Richard, 258

Generation effect, the, 178
Goals, 25, 98, 141, 182–183. *See also* Change goals
Gollwitzer, Peter, 180
Gordon, Thomas, 249
Gorscak, Bonnie, personal change experience of,
　　139–142, 156

Halfhearted action, 167–168
Hurdles, 181–182, 207–211, 227–228, 238

Intention to change, 88, 123, 166
Implementation intentions, 180
Importance of change, 8, 28–30, 33–34, 47, 93–99,
　　103–117, 123–124, 136, 161, 166
　　as a dimension of motivation for change, 30,
　　　34, 89
　　exploring, 103–115
　　confidence for change and, 123–124
　　in motivational interviewing, 252
　　rating, 30–33, 89–92, 98, 115–117
Importance of staying the same (status quo), 86,
　　98–103, 114
　　confidence for change and, 98–99

John (case example), 142–143

Kylie (case example), 140

Leaning toward change, 168–172
Life goals, 185–187, 230
Listening to yourself, 8, 85–86, 88–89, 141–142, 160
Loberg, Kristin, 258
Lost Art of Listening, The (book), 258

Miller, William R., 8, 72, 143, 249–254, 258
MINT Bulletin, 250
Missing pieces of the puzzle, 191–192, 213
Mobilizing talk, 86–88, 166–167
Motivation for change (being motivated), 2, 3, 28,
　　30, 34, 89, 167, 179, 180, 204, 229, 235, 238,
　　239, 246
　　confidence for change as a dimension of, 8,
　　　28–34, 89
　　importance of change as a dimension of, 8,
　　　28–34, 47, 89

Motivational interviewing (MI), 2–3, 7–9, 72, 86,
　　168, 257–258
　　history of, 249–256
　　mechanisms of action, 253
　　midwife analogy, 3
　　personalized feedback in, 252, 254
　　processes in, 252
　　research on, 2, 2n, 252–256
　　spirit of, 9, 252
Motivational Interviewing: Helping People Change
　　(book), 251, 258
*Motivational Interviewing: Preparing People for
　　Change* (book), 251
*Motivational Interviewing: Preparing People to Change
　　Addictive Behavior* (book), 251
*Motivational Interviewing Skills: A Practitioner
　　Workbook* (book), 258
*Motivational Interviewing: Training, Research,
　　Implementation, Practice* (online journal),
　　258
Motivational Interviewing Network of Trainers
　　(MINT), 250, 255–256, 257–258
　　website, 257
Motivational Interviewing with Problem Drinkers
　　(article), 250
Motivational speakers, 42
Moyers, Theresa, 254

Need talk, 87, 92, 98, 102
Neff, Kristin, 62, 258
Neuroimaging, 255
Nichols, Michael P., 258
Norcross, John C., 258
Norcross, Jonathan, 258

On Becoming A Person (book), 249

Parent Effectiveness Training (book), 249
Partnership, 9. *See also* Collaboration
Pathways to change, 232–243
Patterson, Gerald R., 249
Person-centered counseling, 249. *See also* Client-
　　centered counseling
Personal change plan, 8, 138, 164–165, 172, 177,
　　178–180, 181–212
　　commitment to, 211
　　"fit" and, 4, 178, 179, 199, 212
　　goals in, 181, 182–184, 221–222
　　hurdles in, 181–182, 207–211, 212
　　reasons in, 181, 184–188, 222
　　　life goals, 185–187, 230
　　revisiting, 221–228, 234, 238,
　　role of experts in, 178–179
　　steps in, 181, 188–203, 212, 223–224
　　　brainstorming, 194–197, 199
　　　looking back from an ideal future, 197–198
　　　past experience, 190–192
　　　successes and strengths, 192–193
　　signs of success, 228–230
　　support in, 181, 203–207, 212, 225–226

Personal values. *See* Values
Persuasion to change, 3, 5, 6, 7
Pessimism, 119, 123
Positive Qualities You Might Possess (list), 72–73
Preparatory talk, 86–88, 166
Pressure to change
  acceptance and, 63, 82
  anxiety and, 6, 40, 46–47
  avoidance and, 7
  buyer's remorse and, 42
  coercion and, 7
  confrontation and, 6,7
  control and, 37, 39, 47, 57, 62
  defiance of, 6, 40
  defensiveness and, 42
  denial and, 36
  from inside, 7–8, 35–39, 46–58, 170
  from others. *See* from outside
  from outside, 5–8, 35–46, 57–58
  from self. *See* from inside
  guilt and, 6, 7, 41, 47
  helplessness and, 6, 7, 41, 47
  minimization and, 6,7
  negative judgment and, 37, 39, 47, 57, 62
  on self. *See* from inside
  reactance and, 38–39, 246
  readiness to change and, 43
  relief and, 41–42
  sadness and, 41
  shame and, 6, 7, 36, 41, 46–47
  take(ing) the pressure off, 58, 61–63, 65, 71, 82, 170, 217
  threats and, 5,6
Pressure paradox, the, 35, 61–63
Prochaska, James O., 258
Project MATCH, 252–253
Pseudoagreement, 5. *See also* Bobblehead effect
Psychotherapist, 257

Randomized controlled trial (RCT), 253
Reactance, 38–39, 246, 251
  defined, 38
Readiness to change, 89, 138, 164–166, 172
  rating, 165–166
Reason talk, 87, 92, 98, 102
Relationship decision, 2, 13, 15–17, 21, 59–61, 123–124, 185, 236–237, 241–243
Resolve, 166–167
Revisiting your plan, 221–228, 234, 238
Rogers, Carl, 249
Rokeach, Milton, 143
Rollnick, Stephen, 8–9, 72, 251–252
Rosengren, David B., 258
Rosenthal, Robert, 203

Sara (case example), 123–124
Science and Human Behavior (book), 249
Second nature, changes becoming, 207, 235
Self-acceptance, 71, 88, 89, 258
Self-blame, 25–27, 61, 71, 82, 217, 241

Self-compassion, 62, 71, 82, 88, 258. *See also* Compassion
Self-efficacy, 118–119, 188, 251. *See also* Confidence for change
Self-esteem, 28, 30, 37, 143, 258
Self-fulfilling prophecies, 203–204
Self-observation, 215–221
Self-perception theory, 85, 88, 251
Self-rewards, 243–244, 245–247
Self-talk, 47–48
Setbacks, 240–241, 244
Shame, 6, 7, 24, 36, 41, 46–47, 71
Sheila (case example), 59–61, 99
Signs of success, 228–230
Skinner, B.F., 249
Spirit of MI. *See* Motivational interviewing, spirit of
Strengths, 8, 9, 71, 123, 131–134, 178, 192–193
Status quo, 57, 86, 167
  importance of, 98–103, 114
  needs met by, 170–171
Steps toward change, 181, 188–203, 212, 223–224, 234
Successes, 192–193
Support for change, 181, 203–207, 212, 225–226
Sustain talk
  ability talk in, 86–87
  activation talk in, 87, 167
  ambivalence and, 88, 101
  balance of, 98, 123
  commitment talk in, 87, 167
  defined, 86
  desire talk in, 86, 102
  identifying, 95–98, 121–122, 125
  mobilizing talk and, 86–88, 167
  need talk in, 87, 102
  preparatory talk and, 86–88
  reasons talk in, 87, 102
  taking steps talk in, 87, 167

Taking steps talk
  in change talk, 87, 166
  in sustain talk, 87, 167
Terrible triad of ambivalence, 25–27, 82, 241
"There's a Hole in My Bucket" (song), 175–177
Transtheoretical model, 258

Values, 8, 9, 29, 89, 136, 140–161, 172, 185
  conflicting, 142–143

Weight loss, 2, 20–21, 22, 28, 32, 87, 170, 179, 182, 238–240
Why We Do What We Do (book), 258
Worstward Ho (play), 213
Worth, 9, 37

"Yes, but" statements, 5, 7

Zuckoff, Allan, personal change experience of, 231–232

About the Authors

Allan Zuckoff, PhD, is a psychologist who conducts professional training in motivational interviewing (MI) throughout the United States and internationally. He also works to develop new applications of MI for people facing a variety of personal challenges and life issues. Dr. Zuckoff is a member of the international Motivational Interviewing Network of Trainers (MINT) and a faculty member in the Departments of Psychology and Psychiatry at the University of Pittsburgh.

Bonnie Gorscak, PhD, is a psychologist and MI practitioner who has worked in the mental health field for 30 years.